A DEVOTIONAL COMPANION

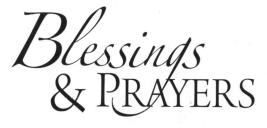

Blessings
& PRAYERS
FOR CAREGIVERS

By Annetta Dellinger and Karen Boerger

CONCORDIA PUBLISHING HOUSE · SAINT LOUIS

Published by Concordia Publishing House, 3558 S. Jefferson Avenue, St. Louis, MO, 63118-3968
1-800-325-3040 • www.cph.org

Text © 2010 Annetta Dellinger and Karen Boerger

Unless otherwise indicated, Scripture quotations are from the ESV Bible® (The Holy Bible, English Standard Version®), copyright © 2001 by Crossway Bibles, a publishing ministry of Good News Publishers. Used by permission. All rights reserved.

Scripture quotations marked NIV are taken from the HOLY BIBLE, NEW INTERNATIONAL VERSION®. NIV®. Copyright © 1973, 1978, 1984 by International Bible Society. Used by permission of Zondervan Publishing House. All rights reserved.

Quotations and hymn texts with the abbreviation LSB are from Lutheran Service Book, copyright © 2006 Concordia Publishing House. All rights reserved.

Orders for Daily Prayer on pages 8–16 are from are from Lutheran Service Book, copyright © 2006 Concordia Publishing House. All rights reserved.

Quotation on page 41 is from Lutheran Service Book: Altar Book, copyright © 2006 Concordia Publishing House. All rights reserved.

Quotations marked Small Catechism are from Luther's Small Catechism with Explanation, copyright © 1986, 1991 Concordia Publishing House. All rights reserved.

All Portals of Prayer quotations are copyright © Concordia Publishing House. All rights reserved.

Quotations on pages 25, 41, and 44 are from Blessings and Prayers for Women: A Devotional Companion, copyright © 2004 Concordia Publishing House. All rights reserved.

Quotations on pages 25, 26, 32, 37, and 40 are from Words of Promise: Daily Devotions through the Year, copyright © 1996 Concordia Publishing House. All rights reserved.

Quotations marked AGPS on pages 30, 31, 32, and 37 are from All God's People Sing!, copyright © 1992 Concordia Publishing House. All rights reserved.

The poem "Strength Warm-Up" on page 78 is © Diana Schnack. Used by permission.

A Brief Summary of the Christian Faith quotations are from Luther's Small Catechism with Explanation, copyright © 1986, 1991 Concordia Publishing House. All rights reserved.

Cover photographs © FreezeFrameStudio and Andrew Howe/iStockphoto.com

Manufactured in the United States of America

Library of Congress Cataloging-in-Publication Data

Dellinger, Annetta E.

Blessings and prayers for caregivers : a devotional companion / by Annetta Dellinger and Karen Boerger.
    p. cm.
    ISBN 978-0-7586-1868-9
1. Caregivers--Prayers and devotions. I. Boerger, Karen. II. Title.
BV4910.9.D45 2009
242'.4--dc22   2009038317

Table of Contents

Preface / Introduction

Dear Caregiver,

Most people have been a caregiver, will become one, or are one right now. There are approximately sixty-five million caregivers in the United States today. You are not alone. Your current circumstances, however, may cause you to feel that you are. Each day can be physically demanding and mentally overwhelming.

As Christians, we don't like to admit to having feelings of loneliness, guilt, anger, sadness, frustration, family conflict, and the like. We want to keep them in a box with the lid fastened down tightly. But when we become caregivers, the lid on the box comes off, and we feel those emotions run rampant throughout our hearts and bodies. There is no putting the lid back on.

So how do we survive? How can we manage these emotions that encircle us twenty-four hours a day, seven days a week? We must find a way to continue to exist in this season of life because our loved ones are counting on us.

- Each morning, ask God to help you and to walk with you on your journey for the day. You are never alone. He is always with you, walking with you, listening to you twenty-four hours a day, seven days a week.

- Next, take care of yourself. Keep healthy foods and snacks available. Don't load up on so-called comfort foods. Exercise and stretch to keep your blood circulating. Confide in your best friend. Tell him or her everything. Encouragement and support are invaluable.

- Always take time for devotions and conversations with your Creator. No, you can't put the lid back on the box, but you can lay your emotional challenges at the foot of the cross. Leave them there, and don't pick them up again. Your Father is quite capable of handling them for you.

This little book provides you with readings of affirmation and encouragement. Prayers, Scriptures, Psalms, and hymns were selected to help you focus on Jesus Christ as the source of all hope, on the strength of God's Holy Word for us, and on the certainty of His promises of mercy, grace, and salvation. *Blessings and Prayers for Caregivers* can be tucked in a pocket or a purse to go with you wherever you are and to be at your fingertips whenever you have a minute or two and need a word of encouragement. And every word was chosen or written from the hearts of those who have been where you are right now.

Blessings and hugs to you and to all the silent heroes who give care to their loved ones!

Annetta Dellinger
Karen Boerger
July, 2009

PRAYERS

Daily Prayer

MORNING

The sign of the cross ✝ may be made in remembrance of your Baptism.

In the name of the Father and of the ✝ Son and of the Holy Spirit.
Amen.

In the morning, O Lord, You hear my voice;
in the morning I prepare a sacrifice for You and watch.

Psalm 5:3

My mouth is filled with Your praise,
and with Your glory all the day.

Psalm 71:8

O Lord, open my lips,
and my mouth will declare Your praise.

Psalm 51:15

Glory be to the Father and to the Son and to the Holy Spirit;
as it was in the beginning, is now, and will be forever. Amen.

A hymn, canticle, or psalm may be sung or spoken.

An appointed reading or one of the following is read: Colossians 3:1–4;

Exodus 15:1–11; Isaiah 12:1–6; Matthew 20:1–16; Mark 13:32–36; Luke 24:1–9; John 21:4–14; Ephesians 4:17–24; Romans 6:1–4.

A portion of the Small or Large Catechism may be read.

The Apostles' Creed is confessed.

Lord's Prayer

Prayers for others and ourselves

Concluding prayers:

Almighty God, merciful Father, who created and completed all things, on this day when the work of our calling begins anew, we implore You to create its beginning, direct its continuance, and bless its end, that our doings may be preserved from sin, our life sanctified, and our work this day be well pleasing to You; through Jesus Christ, our Lord.
Amen.

I thank You, my heavenly Father, through Jesus Christ, Your dear Son, that You have kept me this night from all harm and danger; and I pray that You would keep me this day also from sin and every evil, that all my doings in life may please You. For into Your hands I commend myself, my body and soul, and all things. Let Your holy angel be with

me, that the evil foe may have no power over me. Amen. (423)

Let us bless the Lord.
Thanks be to God.

Now go joyfully to your work.

(*LSB*, p. 295)

Noon Prayer

The sign of the cross + may be made in remembrance of your Baptism.

In the name of the Father and of the ✝ Son and of the Holy Spirit.
Amen.

Listen to my prayer, O God, do not ignore my plea;
hear me and answer me.

Evening, morning, and noon
I cry out in distress, and He hears my voice.

Cast your cares on the Lord and He will sustain you;
He will never let the righteous fall.

Psalm 55:1–2a, 17, 22 NIV

Glory be to the Father and to the Son and to the Holy Spirit;
as it was in the beginning, is now, and will be forever. Amen.

A hymn, canticle, or psalm may be sung or spoken.

An appointed reading or one of the following is read: 1 Corinthians 7:17a, 23–24; Luke 23:44–46; Matthew 5:13–16; Matthew 13:1–9, 18–23; Mark 13:24–27; John 15:1–9; Romans 7:18–25; Romans 12:1–2; 1 Peter 1:3–9; Revelation 7:13–17.

O Lord,
have mercy upon us.

O Christ,
have mercy upon us.

O Lord,
have mercy upon us. Mark 10:47

Lord's Prayer

Prayers for others and ourselves

Concluding prayer:

Blessed Lord Jesus Christ, at this hour You hung upon the cross, stretching out Your loving arms to embrace the world in Your death. Grant that all people of the earth may look to You and see their salvation; for Your mercy's sake we pray.
Amen.

Heavenly Father, send Your Holy Spirit into our hearts to direct and rule us according to Your will, to comfort us in all our afflictions, to defend us form all error, and to lead us into all truth; through Jesus Christ, our Lord.

Amen.

Let us bless the Lord.
Thanks be to God.   [Psalm 103:1]

(*LSB*, p. 296)

EARLY EVENING

The sign of the cross ✝ may be made in remembrance of your Baptism.

In the name of the Father and of the ✝ Son and of the Holy Spirit.
Amen.

A candle may be lighted.

Let my prayer rise before You as incense,
the lifting up of my hands as the evening sacrifice.   Psalm 141:2

Joyous light of glory:
of the immortal Father;
heavenly, holy, blessed Jesus Christ.
We have come to the setting of the sun,
and we look to the evening light.
We sing to God, the Father, Son, and Holy Spirit:
You are worthy of being praised with pure voices forever.
O Son of God, O Giver of life: the universe proclaims Your glory.

A hymn, canticle, or psalm may be sung or spoken.

An appointed reading or one of the following is read: Luke 24:28–31; Exodus 16:11–21, 31; Isaiah 25:6–9; Matthew 14:15–21; Matthew 27:57–60; Luke 14:15–24; John 6:25–35; John 10:7–18; Ephesians 6:10–18a.

A portion of the Small or Large Catechism may be read.

Lord's Prayer

Prayers for others and ourselves

Concluding prayer:

Lord Jesus, stay with us, for the evening is at hand and the day is past. Be our constant companion on the way, kindle our hearts, and awaken hope among us, that we may recognize You as You are revealed in the Scriptures and in the breaking of the bread. Grant this for Your name's sake. **Amen.**

Let us bless the Lord.
Thanks be to God. [Psalm 103:1]

(*LSB*, p. 297)

MEALTIME PRAYERS

Asking a blessing before the meal

Lord God, heavenly Father, bless us and these

Your gifts which we receive from Your bountiful goodness, through Jesus Christ, our Lord. Amen.

(*LSB*, p. 297)

Returning thanks after the meal

We thank You, Lord God, heavenly Father, for all Your benefits, through Jesus Christ, our Lord, who lives and reigns with You and the Holy Spirit forever and ever. Amen.

(*LSB*, p. 297)

CLOSE OF THE DAY

The sign of the cross ✝ may be made in remembrance of your Baptism.

In the name of the Father and of the ✝ Son and of the Holy Spirit.
Amen.

The Lord Almighty grant us a quiet night and peace at the last.
Amen.

It is good to give thanks to the Lord,
to sing praise to Your name, O Most High;

To herald Your love in the morning,
Your truth at the close of the day.

An appointed reading or one of the following is read: Matthew 11:28–30; Micah 7:18–20; Matthew 18:15–35; Matthew 25:1–13;

Luke 11:1–13; Luke 12:13–34; Romans 8:31–39; 2 Corinthians 4:16–18; Revelation 21:22–22:5.

The Apostles' Creed is confessed.

Lord, now You let Your servant go in peace;
  Your word has been fulfilled.
My own eyes have seen the salvation
  which You have prepared in the sight of
    every people:
A light to reveal You to the nations
  and the glory of Your people Israel.

Luke 2:29–32

Glory be to the Father and to the Son and to
  the Holy Spirit;
as it was in the beginning, is now, and will
  be forever. Amen.

Lord's Prayer

Prayers for others and ourselves

Concluding prayers:

Visit our dwellings, O Lord, and in Your great mercy defend us from all perils and dangers of this night; for the love of Your only Son, our Savior Jesus Christ.
Amen.

I thank You, my heavenly Father, through Jesus Christ, Your dear Son, that You have graciously kept me this day; and I pray that You would forgive me all my sins where I have done wrong, and graciously keep me this night. For into Your hands I commend myself, my body and my soul, and all things. Let Your holy angel be with me, that the evil foe may have no power over me. Amen.

Let us bless the Lord. [Psalm 103:1]
Thanks be to God.

Then go to sleep at once and in good cheer.

(*LSB*, p. 298)

General Prayers

THE LORD'S PRAYER

Our Father who art in heaven,

hallowed be Thy name,

Thy kingdom come,

Thy will be done on earth as it is in heaven;

give us this day our daily bread;

and forgive us our trespasses as we forgive
those who trespass against us;

and lead us not into temptation,

but deliver us from evil,

For Thine is the kingdom and the power and the
glory forever and ever. Amen.

LUTHER'S MORNING PRAYER

I thank You, my heavenly Father, through Jesus Christ, Your dear Son, that You have kept me this night from all harm and danger; and I pray that You would keep me this day also from sin and every evil, that all my doings and life may please You. For into Your hands I commend myself, my body and soul, and all things. Let Your holy angel be with me, that the evil foe may have no power over me. Amen.

(*Small Catechism*, p. 33)

Luther's Evening Prayer

I thank You, my heavenly Father, through Jesus Christ, Your dear Son, that You have graciously kept me this day; and I pray that You would forgive me all my sins where I have done wrong, and graciously keep me this night. For into Your hands I commend myself, my body and soul, and all things. Let Your holy angel be with me, that the evil foe may have no power over me. Amen.

(Small Catechism, p. 33)

Sunday

It's a great day to have been with You in worship, Lord. Give Your Holy Spirit to all who approached Your altar to eat and drink the body and blood of Your dear Son. Thank you for the precious gifts of Your Word and Sacrament. Comfort all who mourn or are heavy laden. Give patience to the sick and hurting, and wisdom to the doctors and nurses who care for them. Forgive my sins for the sake of Your Son's suffering, and grant me Your mercy as You promised. In His name, Amen.

(Adapted from Portals of Prayer, April–June 2009, p. 98)

Monday

Father, it's the beginning of a new week. Thank You for the refreshment of the weekend, both for the bodily rest and the spiritual food of Your Word. Thank You also for granting me another day that I may serve You in caring for my loved one. Be with me as we face each new challenge together and give me joy as I accomplish each task placed before me. Whether this day brings happiness or sadness, let me draw my strength from You. Help me to be slow to anger, quick to forgive, and willing to serve You by serving others. In Your name I pray. Amen.

TUESDAY

Lord Jesus, one night in Gethsemane, the forces of evil gathered to attack You. You prayed intently while Your disciples fell into sleep, unable to keep watch with You. Later, You deepened their faith. Make us worthy of the calling You have given us. Fill us with Your grace and gifts, granting us a patient, gentle love for one another, that together, we may be faithful servants through whom You build Your kingdom. As You came to the disciples after Your resurrection to relieve their fear, relieve our fears by Your Word. Send Your angels to watch over us, keeping us in Your perfect love. In Your name we pray. Amen.

(*Portals of Prayer*, July–September 2008, p. 101)

Wednesday

My faithful God, I thank You for the grace, mercy, and peace from You, Father, and from Jesus Christ, Your Son, that are with me in truth and love. I humble myself before You and trust that You will lift me up. Send me encouragers when I need them, and quiet and rest when I'm overwhelmed. Every day I am in need of Your grace, so help me maintain an attitude that welcomes it. Grant me Your peace through Jesus Christ, our Lord. Amen.

Thursday

God, as one of Your chosen people, holy and dearly loved, help me to clothe myself with compassion, kindness, humility, gentleness, and patience. Please give me an attitude the same as that of Christ Jesus. Help me to sense Your presence in my life. I need You more than I can say. Help me, Lord, not to be anxious about anything, but in everything, by prayer and supplication, with thanksgiving, to present my requests to You. And Your peace, O God, which transcends all understanding, will guard my heart and my mind in Christ Jesus. Amen.

Friday

Gracious God, You have brought me to the beginning of this new day in the name of the Father and the Son and the Holy Spirit. Strengthen me by Your Word so that I will have courage to face temptation and grace to overcome it. Keep me from sin and every evil. Help me represent You well in all the places I go today. Prepare me to tell someone today of the hope that is within me because of the death and resurrection of Jesus and His love for me. Lead me to speak with gentleness and reverence. For all this, I praise You, O God, for You are my Rock and my Redeemer. In the name of the Lord Jesus Christ, I pray. Amen.

(*Portals of Prayer*, January–March 2009, p. 102)

Saturday

Thank You, Lord, for this day to spend with family and friends. Grant us refreshing times that strengthen our bodies and renew our spirits. The list is long of all we hope to accomplish this weekend. We have homes to care for, yards to tend, and other chores that need to be done. The requests for our time are many. Family, friends, community, and church all need us. Help us fill the days with productive labor and meaningful time with those we love and those who need us. Help and guide us so that, by the end of the day, we will have used

Your gifts in meaningful ways that reflect Your love and our faith in You. Amen.

(*Portals of Prayer*, July–September 2009, p. 105)

Morning

It's a new day, heavenly Father, and I know there is nothing You and I can't handle together. Help me to stay focused on my caregiving duties so that by evening I can look back and say I have been able to glorify You. During this day, let me praise You for what You have created and the blessings You have bestowed. You are the true light that sustains me. Let Your light so shine in my life that others unknown to me see it and give You praise. In the name of Jesus, Amen.

Midday

Most gracious Father, it was at this hour that Your Son hung upon the cross, offering His life for the salvation of the world. Thank You for His sacrifice, which atoned for all our sins. We rejoice that through Baptism, You have joined us to His death and resurrection. Grant that, recalling His death and remembering our own Baptism, we would daily die to sin and rise to newness of life. Be with us and strengthen us for the tasks that remain to be accomplished this day. Help us reflect Your love in all that we say and do, and draw us ever back to You, even amid the busyness of today. In Jesus' name we pray. Amen.

(*Portals of Prayer*, January–March 2009, p. 104)

EVENING

Merciful Father, what a joy to come to You this evening. As this day comes to a close, we thank You for Your blessings of body and soul. Give us a restful night that we may rise in the morning ready for the Word of God to refresh us. Give us gracious hearts toward those who fail us, hearts formed and fashioned by the grace You have shown us in Your Son, Jesus. In His name we pray, Amen.

BEFORE MEALS

Come, Lord Jesus, be our guest and let these gifts to us be blessed. Amen.

Lord God, heavenly Father, bless us and these Your gifts which we receive from Your bountiful goodness, through Jesus Christ, our Lord. Amen.

(*Small Catechism*, p. 34)

AFTER MEALS

Oh, give thanks unto the Lord for He is good, for His mercy endures forever. Amen.

Topical Prayers

ASSURANCE

Father, You have called Your servants to ventures of which we can see neither the end nor the unknown challenges ahead. Give us assurance that what we do is pleasing to You. Give us faith to go out with good courage, not knowing where we go, but only that Your hand is leading us and Your love supporting us, through Jesus Christ our Lord. Amen.

BIRTHDAY

Faithful Father, thank You for another year of Your tender mercies and faithful provision. I praise You for Your constant presence in both the heartaches and the joys of the past year. Help me rely on Your grace and leave my guilt, worries, and doubts behind. Equip me through Your Word to press forward toward knowing You more fully and becoming more like You in thought, action, and purpose. Amen.

(Portals of Prayer, April–June 2008, p. 114)

By a Hospice Worker

Almighty God, heavenly Father, as You have taken my life and made it holy in the death of Your Son, Jesus Christ, so, too, take the labor of my hands into Your own holy hands to accomplish Your will. Strengthen me in my work so discouragement, anger, and sadness do not overtake me, but that all I do may be pleasing in Your sight; through Jesus Christ, Your Son, our Lord. Amen.

(Adapted from Blessings and Prayers for Women,
p. 155, prayer 41)

By One Who Is Ill

Merciful Father, I come to You, acknowledging my sin and unworthiness. Still I trust Your promise for Jesus' sake to hear my prayer and to give me whatever needful blessings I ask in His name. I implore You to lay Your healing hand on me. Add Your blessing to the ministrations of doctors and nurses and to the medicine that I am receiving during this time of my illness. If it be Your will, renew and restore my health and strength. I commend myself into Your gracious care and keeping. I ask that through the presence and power of Your Holy Spirit You would keep me strong in faith. Grant this for Jesus' sake. Amen.

(Words of Promise, p. 337)

I'm depressed, dear Lord, and I'm tired of being sick. When I think of all the things I could and should be doing, I get discouraged. Lord Jesus, You understand what suffering and pain are like. Thank You for enduring misery and agony to free me from the burden of my sins. Thank You for loving me. Thank You for providing people to help me. Renew their strength. Lord, keep me from complaining so much that I turn others away. Help me to show those around me that I'm confident in Your love. Only You can heal me, Lord. If it is Your will, make me well. I believe, Lord. Increase my faith. Amen.

(*Words of Promise*, p. 339)

CAREGIVERS

Lord, we pray for those who serve others as caregivers, that they may exhibit Your care. Let them be Your hands in administering Your love, whether they serve children, the mentally or physically impaired, or the elderly. Strengthen them when their responsibilities are heavy. When those whom they serve lack gratitude, let them find joy in knowing that in serving others they are serving You. Amen.

(*Portals of Prayer*, April–June 2008, p. 111)

CHILDREN

O Lord, our merciful Shepherd, graciously regard the little lambs of Your dear flock, especially the young, that they might not fall away from Your flock, but grow constantly in grace and wisdom. Be their constant guide and companion. Instill in them both a steadfast faith and a love for virtue. Teach them to abhor evil and to shun falsehood. And guard them from every evil of body and soul. Amen.

(*Portals of Prayer*, July–September 2008, p. 109)

DEATH

Prior to a Loved One's Death

O God, my loved one is nearing the time of death. Help me to speak words of assurance to him or her as well as to provide caring comfort that will help him or her rest well. He or she has been my companion for many years and has been a blessing and inspiration to me. I am glad that he or she knows You and Your saving grace through Your Son, Jesus Christ. I take comfort in the Scripture verse, "We know that the one who raised the Lord Jesus from the dead will also raise us with Jesus" (2 Corinthians 4:14). I commend my loved one to You now. I also ask You to comfort and strengthen me during this difficult time. In Jesus' name. Amen.

After a Loved One's Death

O God, I am filled with deep grief and loss. My loved one and I went through the caregiving journey together, and even though I was expecting this, it's still very difficult to know that he or she is gone. Comfort me, and give me strength to fill the emptiness in my life. Fill me with Your peace and love. Receive my loved one into Your glorious kingdom so that he or she may rest in Your love, peace, and joy forever. In Jesus' name. Amen

DIFFICULT DECISION

Dear Father, we made the difficult decision that it's time for our loved one to move into a care facility. It wasn't easy, but we did it. We thank You for the professional caregivers in his or her new home. Fill them with Your Spirit so they respond to our loved one competently and compassionately. Bless our loved one as he or she adjusts to the new home. Fill us with Your peace today and every day. We need You. In Jesus' name we pray. Amen.

DISCOURAGED

Heavenly Father, You are my refuge and strength. I am so tired and discouraged, but then I remember that You are not a stranger to discouragement and suffering. You understand, and I am uplifted to know You care for me. Your strength comforts me. Help me find peace once more. Continue to care and to show Your love for me so that I may show Your love to my loved one. In Jesus Christ, Your Son, our Lord. Amen.

FOR THE DISABLED

Lord God, heavenly Father, we thank You for the gift of life and everything in Your creation that enriches our physical lives. By Your merciful guidance, aid and strengthen those with physical disabilities, and enable them to find fulfillment in their lives and encouragement and support for all their endeavors; through Jesus Christ, our Lord. [Amen.]

(LSB, p. 317)

FEAR

Dear heavenly Father, be my guide and comforter. Help me to be content in knowing You and Your love. Be near me when I suffer the "whys" of life. Assure me of Your constant love and care for me. Continue to warm me with Your love in Christ as I face the challenges ahead. In His name. Amen.

Father, help me to overcome my fears. Remind me that You are my constant shepherd and keep me in Your care so I will not be in want or wander in life's valleys. Fill my heart with Your peace and use my hands for Your service. In Jesus' name. Amen.

"I am trusting Thee, Lord Jesus, trusting only Thee" (*LSB*, 729). As I remember the quiet trust of peaceful days in my life, I know it has prepared me for the storms of life that I'm feeling right now. Guide me, support me, and hold my hand as together we walk through the challenges of this life together. In Jesus Christ, Amen.

For God's Word

Dear heavenly Father, You have given us a great gift in Your Holy Word. Make us attentive as we listen to it and study it. Make clear for us Your will for our lives. Hear us for Jesus' sake. Amen.

(*AGPS*, p. 32)

For Long-Distance Caregiving

Heavenly Father, I thank You for the care my loved one is receiving. He or she needs our special care but lives so far away from me. Guide me so I can be a loving and effective caregiver even at this distance—and give me the energy to do so.

Guide all my thoughts, words, and deeds so I can be a blessing to him or her. Minister to my feelings of guilt for not being there constantly. Fill me with Your love, guidance, and peace. In Jesus' name I pray. Amen.

For My Loved One in My Care

Lord Jesus, look upon me in Your mercy and grant me Your help. Give me a patient and cheerful spirit. Draw my heart heavenward to think about Your love for me. Grant me the peace of salvation that You have purchased for me with Your blood. Guide me in the paths of righteousness that I may walk with You and be a willing servant for my loved one. Bless *(name)*, who is in my care, so Your compassion for him or her fills his or her heart with the peace and comfort that only You can give. Extend Your healing hand to all those who are ill. I pray this in Your name. Amen.

For the Sick

Lord Jesus, our Creator and Keeper, we remember *(name)* who is sick (hurt). Be with those who tend to him (her). Strengthen his (her) family and friends in this time. Remind them of Your great love and care for us. If it be Your will, restore to them sound health of body, soul, and mind. Hear our prayer for Your name's sake. Amen.

(*AGPS*, p. 32)

Lord Jesus Christ, we know You have pity on the sick. We remember that while You walked the roads of Palestine You cured the deaf, the blind, the lame, and the lepers. Help us to believe You are present now in a very real way. Lord Jesus, look in mercy on *(names)*. Reach out Your gracious hand and grant a healing. Increase the wisdom and skill of doctors and nurses who minister to the sick as Your instruments. Use us to demonstrate Your love in cheering, visiting, and caring for the sick. Above all, we ask for spiritual healing for the sick and for us through Your Word. Amen.

(*Words of Promise*, p. 325)

For Sharing the Word

Dear Lord, You are our Savior and King. You always forgive us when we do wrong or fail to do what is right. Keep us humble, trusting in Your grace and mercy. But make us bold too; bold to live for You by serving others, bold to speak Your Word, bold to be known as Christians wherever we go. Teach us those truths You want us to know. We pray in Jesus' name. Amen.

(*AGPS*, p. 33)

Forgiveness

Lord Jesus, thank You for caring about how much I have been hurt. You know the pain I have felt because of *(list each offense)*. Right now I release all that pain into Your hands. Thank You, Lord, for dying on the cross for me and extending Your forgiveness to me. As an act of my will, I choose to forgive *(name)*. I take him or her off my emotional hook and transfer it all to You. I refuse all thoughts of revenge. And Lord, thank You for giving me Your power to forgive so I can be set free. In Your name and for Your sake, I pray. Amen.

Future

Eternal God, we ask Your presence and blessing on our future days. We implore You to pardon the sins we have committed. Help us to remember You daily. Please guide us in all our ways. Guard and keep us under Your protection, so that we may live our lives in Your grace and peace. In Christ's name we pray. Amen.

Grief

As I grieve, O God, help me to express my feelings. Grief is not easy, and I sometimes forget or become confused. I'm told this is normal, but when will my *real* normal return? Help me to get proper rest, eat nutritiously, and exercise. These are things that I was told to do during my caregiving days, but I am having trouble doing them now. Comfort me, Lord, with Your love and fill me with the peace that I know only You can give. This I pray in Jesus' name. Amen.

Guidance

Lord, because You know everything, You know the decision before me and the way I should go. I want only Your will, Lord. I no longer have the option of waiting, so I will choose (*one of the options*). If this decision is not right in Your sight, I ask Your Holy Spirit to put a heaviness in my heart. If this is the right direction for me to take, please confirm it with Your peace. I am willing to take whatever detours You decide to put in my path, as long as I reach the destination You have for me. I am in Your hands. In Christ's precious name I pray. Amen.

Guilt

Heavenly Father, I confess my sin of _____ _____ to You, and I am willing to turn from it. Thank You for Your forgiveness. I will rely on the power of Christ within me to overcome my times of temptation. Thank You for Your grace and mercy toward me. In Jesus' name I pray. Amen.

Oh, God, Your Word speaks to me. Psalm 40:2 says, "He drew me up from the pit of destruction, out of the miry bog, and set my feet upon a rock, making my steps secure." My feet were definitely in the miry bog today, Lord. I was frustrated and became angry, but the worst part of it was that I let my loved one see my anger. Forgive me, Lord, and help me to forgive myself. Be with me as I continue my caregiving duties and help me to always set my feet upon a rock, especially the rock of Your salvation. In Jesus Christ, our Lord. Amen.

HEALING

Lord Jesus, during Your earthly ministry, You healed many, demonstrating that You are the Savior of both body and soul. Lord, I pray for those who are sick and suffering. Grant them healing according to Your good and gracious will. Bless the doctors, nurses, and caregivers who serve them. Amid their illness, enable them to trust in Your all-sufficient grace and to rejoice in Your strength, even in their time of weakness. In Your name I pray. Amen.

(*Portals of Prayer*, January–March, 2009, p. 114)

Heavenly Father, You are the Creator and Giver of life and health. Look in mercy upon all who are suffering in both mind and body. Show Your love to the handicapped and infirm. Be with the aged and those at the point of death. Bless all who minister and care for these people. Let Your healing power restore them to health or ease them in their illnesses. Shower them with Your love and comfort and give them strength that they may bear their afflictions with patience and courage. If it be Your will, heal them that they may serve You with thankfulness. In Jesus' name. Amen.

HOLIDAYS

Heavenly Father, my loved one and our family have had wonderful holidays together in the past. Now, because of our loved one's limitations, I am unsure if we can handle preparing for this occasion. Our memories of the past are heartwarming, but we know it's not the same anymore. Help us to keep a spiritual perspective on this special occasion and upon our relationship. I pray that this holiday will be a time to cherish forever as we create new memories to treasure in our hearts. Bless us with Your love and peace. In Jesus' name we pray. Amen.

HOME/FAMILY

Dear Lord, we give You thanks for the gift of our family. Give us Your kind of love for one another. Help us to be forgiving, kind, and true. Especially we ask that You would keep us close to You. Give us joy in the reading of Your Word and in our times of praising You together. Protect us in times of danger, and keep our trust always in You. Come, Lord Jesus, be our Guest! Amen.

(AGPS, p. 32)

IN THE MIDST OF TRIALS

Lord, we are weak, but You are strong. Give us Your strength to endure the problems of life. Help those who are suffering through illness, from the loss of a loved one, or from emotional problems. Especially we pray for any who are involved in alcoholism, depression, or drug abuse. Keep them and us strong through faith as we continue to look to You, our Rock. Turn our hearts toward You, for You hear our cries for help. Your love sustains us. You lift us and offer us the comfort of Your Word, giving us the power of Your Holy Spirit within us to give us strength. In Jesus' name we pray. Amen.

(Words of Promise, p. 341)

Joy

Dear God, You are *my* caregiver. Sometimes I get so overwhelmed with the daily challenges that I forget to acknowledge You as the one who loves and cares for me. I can relate to Paul because I do the things I don't want to do, and what I want to do—totally focus on You—I don't do. What a relief to know that You will never stop loving me even when I lose my focus and forget that You are the source of my strength. What an inexpressible joy I feel knowing that I will never be helpless as Your child. Your love for me is everlasting. I never have to give up hope. It is with wondrous joy that I praise You for being my caregiver. In Your name. Amen.

"I've got the joy, joy, joy, joy down in my heart!" Thank You, Lord, for the many reasons for joy each day of our lives and especially for the wonderful day my loved one and I shared together. Continue to hold us in Your strength and help us to rejoice in You today, tomorrow, and always. In Your Son's name. Amen.

For Those Who Are Lonely

Ever-present Lord, You have promised never to leave us nor forsake us but to abide with us to the end of time. Grant that those who live alone may not be lonely but find both comfort from Your promises and fulfillment in loving You and their neighbors all their days; through Jesus Christ, our Lord.

(LSB, p. 317)

Gracious God, through Christ, You have promised that You will never leave us or forsake us. Give grace to the lonely, that by Your Word and Spirit, these promises will strengthen them and give heart to their confession, even while loneliness tests their confidence in You. Comfort them through Jesus, who endured the cross alone and forsaken, giving Himself gladly, that even in loneliness, they may be Your children and abide in Your presence. Amen.

(Portals of Prayer, January–March, 2009, p. 116)

Lord Jesus, who experienced absolute loneliness and forsakenness on the cross, send Your Spirit to me as I am feeling lonely today. Speak to me through Your Word, giving me the promise of Your unseen yet everlasting presence. Through the members of Your Body, the Church, make Your presence known through a note, a phone call, or a visit. Uplift me with the truth that because You were forsaken, I never will be. In Your name. Amen.

(Adapted from *Portals of Prayer*, July–September, 2009, p. 117)

"What a friend we have in Jesus, all our sins and griefs to bear!" Thank You for Your presence in my life. Loneliness seems to have grabbed hold of me and won't let go. Sometimes I long for a friend to talk to. Then I remember You are my Friend, and You are always there to listen and give me hope. Forgive me when I don't come to You sooner. Your comforting arms bring peace to my soul and order to my life. Thank You, Lord Jesus, for listening and for helping me face those things that would rob me of faith and joy. Help me to never neglect those precious moments when I can speak to You—alone. Amen.

MEDICAL PROFESSIONALS

Ever-caring Savior, who has carried all our griefs and burdens for us, uphold all those who attend to the needs of others. Give them patience and perseverance when the task seems overwhelming and futile. Help them to see their service as a fruit of the saving faith that Your Holy Spirit has given them. Teach all of us the joy of bearing each other's burdens, thus loving each other as You first loved us. We ask this in Your holy name. Amen.

(Portals of Prayer, April–June 2009, p. 113)

Most merciful Father, You have committed to our love and care our fellow human beings and their necessities. Graciously be with and prosper all those who serve the sick and those in need. Let their service be abundantly blessed as they bring relief to the suffering, comfort to the sorrowing, and peace to the dying. Grant them the knowledge that inasmuch as they do it unto the least of the Master's brethren, they do it unto Him; through the same Jesus Christ, our Lord.

(LSB Altar Book, p. 452)

MERCY

Almighty and everlasting God, always more ready to hear than we to pray and always ready to give more than we either desire or deserve, pour down upon us the abundance of Your mercy, forgiving us those things of which our conscience is afraid, and giving us those good things we are not worthy to ask but through the merits and mediation of Jesus Christ, Your Son, our Lord. Amen.

(Blessings and Prayers for Women, p. 149, prayer 26)

Money/Finances

Heavenly Father, I need Your help. I am humbled in Your presence for You have cleansed me from the stain of my sins. The costs of medical treatments are rising and the frequency of our need for them is mounting. Our fixed income can only be stretched so far. You said in Matthew 6:34, "Therefore do not be anxious about tomorrow, for tomorrow will be anxious for itself. Sufficient for the day is its own trouble." I'm trying to listen and trust You, Lord. Help me to accept my circumstances and to continue to find new paths of financial help. I acknowledge my total dependence on You. In Jesus' name I pray. Amen.

Peace

Lord God, heavenly Father, You sent Your Son to be the Prince of Peace and to give us true and lasting peace in the forgiveness of our sins. Grant me Your peace, the peace the world cannot give, and help me live by faith, to trust in You for all things, to forgive others as You have forgiven me, and to rest confidently in Your love. In Jesus' name. Amen.

(*Portals of Prayer*, October–December 2009, p. 117)

Repentance

Merciful Father, grant us the help of Your divine aid, that we may not fall into temptation or be led in the way of destruction. Look not upon our sins, nor on their account deny our prayer, but lead us into true repentance, that we may truly lament our sins and receive from the depth of Your mercy full pardon of all our transgressions; through the merit of Your Son, our Savior Jesus Christ. Amen.

(Portals of Prayer, July–September 2008, p. 108)

Salvation

God, I want a real relationship with You. I admit that many times I've chosen to go my own way instead of Your way. Please forgive me for my sins. Jesus, thank You for dying on the cross to pay the full penalty for all my sins. Show me my true value in Your eyes. Through Your love and Your power, make me the person You created me to be. In Your holy name I pray. Amen.

Strength

Father, as You helped Your Son as He walked the way of sorrows carrying His cross, comfort and strengthen me as I bear my cross. Keep me from losing faith in this time of testing, and increase my trust in You even more. Help me believe that You are at work through this trial, and cause me to remember "that the sufferings of this present time are not worth comparing with the glory that is to be revealed" (Romans 8:18). I pray in Jesus' name. Amen.

(*Portals of Prayer*, January–March, 2009, p. 110)

Father of all mercy, You never fail to help those who call on You for help. Give strength and confidence to Your servant in my time of great need that I may know that You are near and that underneath me are Your everlasting arms. Grant that, resting in Your protection, I may fear no evil, for You are with me to comfort and deliver me through Jesus Christ, Your Son, our Lord. Amen.

(Adapted from *Blessings and Prayers for Women*, p. 152, prayer 32)

Heavenly Father, help me to trust that for Jesus' sake You will give me the strength needed for each day. Be with me and turn my weakness into strength. Help me to cling to Your Word and rely on Your presence. As I trust in You, grant me victory over weakness and discouragement. In Christ Jesus, Amen.

Father, You are my comforter. You are the reason I get up each morning with a joyful heart. My loved one doesn't know me anymore; therefore, I come to talk to You about all that has happened throughout the day. I know You listen, Lord, and it gives me strength. I am truly grateful. Although I can't always understand Your plan for the future, I trust Your wisdom and guidance. I know that I am loved because of Your dear Son, Jesus, my Savior. Amen.

Shut-ins

Dear Father, comforter of the lonely and hope of the distressed, remember in mercy those who are unable to venture from their homes. Assure them of Your love in Christ through the forgiveness of sins. Grant them confidence and joy in Your promise to be with them always by means of Your Word. Through Christ, who bore the cross for us, let their cross draw them to Your power and love. Strengthen their faith, and help us be their loving neighbors. Amen.

(*Portals of Prayer*, January–March 2009, p. 116)

Merciful Jesus, be with the homebound, especially *(names)*. Give them patience in their limitations. Help them see the honor You give them, for in allowing others to care for them, they become the representatives through whom others serve You (Matthew 25:40). Touch them with Your love and hope through us. Provide them abundant opportunities to receive Your Word and Sacrament. Help them see You at work giving meaning to their lives. Amen.

(*Portals of Prayer*, July–September, 2009, p. 113)

SPOUSE

O God, it is so difficult to adjust to this new marital relationship of being a caregiver to my spouse because he or she needs extra help. I long for the days when we enjoyed doing things together. Now we are together, but it is different. He or she needs a lot of help from me, and I need a lot of help from You and others to care for him or her. You are my refuge from whom I draw strength. I know You care for me, and I ask for Your guidance. Walk with me during this difficult time. In Jesus' name I pray. Amen.

THANKSGIVING

We give You thanks, dear Father, for sending Your Son to make a lifelong journey to save us. When we are given the opportunity to care for loved ones, family, or friends, may we consider it an honor to reach out to them in Your name. Give us cheerful hearts that we may continue to encourage and uplift those we love, helping us to erase doubt or fear. We trust in You and give You thanks. In Jesus' name. Amen.

1 Season of Life
Caregiving—A Season of Life

For everything there is a season, and a time for every matter under heaven. Ecclesiastes 3:1

One morning I discovered a turtledove had built her nest in the crook of the downspout by the patio where I have morning coffee and quiet time with God. As I watched her, she sat steadfastly on her perch and didn't budge.

Morning after morning, Mrs. Dove was there to greet me. We watched each other, each with a different purpose.

During our morning quiet times, I watched this mama bird do one thing and one thing only—rest on her nest, warming and protecting her tiny eggs. She sat, undaunted, even when one day brought a violent storm that blew through with loud claps of thunder, crackling flashes of lightning, and pelting sheets of rain.

On another morning as I was gazing at Mrs. Dove's contented status, I pondered her situation.

She was doing what God had made her to do for this season of her life, and she was *content* and *intent* in doing it. Regardless of storms or the stares of others, she did not move from her task.

If caregiving is now your calling, remember the contentment of the turtledove. God calls us to a constant, living relationship with Him through faith in Christ, our Savior. Through Baptism, we are adopted into the family of believers and assured of eternal life in heaven. Now that's contentment!

Through this season of your life, God, your caregiver, is there beside you. "Fear not, for I am with you; be not dismayed, for I am your God; I will strengthen you, I will help you, I will uphold you with My righteous right hand" (Isaiah 41:10).

Great is His faithfulness!

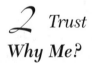

2 Trust

Why Me?

Trust in the LORD with all your heart, and do not lean on your own understanding.
In all your ways acknowledge Him, and He will make straight your paths. Proverbs 3:5–6

"But why?" my granddaughter kept asking. I replied in my grown-up voice, "I know you don't understand. Just trust me."

I can relate to her endless list of questioning *why*. I do that to my heavenly Father. It was not my plan to be a caregiver. I feel like I am exiled from my normal routine that used to make up my day. I miss sleeping in once in a while. I miss my freedom.

God asks us to trust Him even when we do not understand. His grace will bring good out of *all* things, not just some things! Going to Nineveh was not in Jonah's plans. Joseph didn't plan to be abused by his siblings, left in a pit to die, and then imprisoned. But we know that God had a plan for Jonah and for Joseph. God's plan is perfect. Be hope-filled by God's faithfulness!

The good will not erase what you are going through, but never doubt that God's plan is embroidered with the beauty of His mercy in all the colors of His love. God's Word validates the reasons we should not lean on our own understanding. We are to trust in what Jesus did for us on the cross.

Be assured that a season in caregiving is like a season in nature. A season is not necessarily a brief time but it is a limited time. No season lasts forever. "See! The winter is past; . . . Flowers appear on the earth" (Song of Solomon 2:11–12, NIV). What does last forever is that Jesus' death on Good Friday gave way to the joy of Easter morning with His resurrection and promise of eternal life.

Caregiver, take your faith walk one day at a time. Praise God for His "blessings in disguise." Be refreshed as you grow more in love with your Savior, Jesus Christ, as you walk with Him through this season of your life.

God is faithful in all things!

3 Worth
A Caregiver's Real Worth

Even the hairs of your head are all numbered.
Fear not; you are of more value than many sparrows.
Luke 12:7

A weary caregiver recently commented, "I do the same things *every* single day. Dispense medications. Change linens. Do laundry. Suddenly it is time for the next round of pills and a diaper change. I try my best to prepare special dietary meals between being available whenever she calls.

She probably appreciates me, but just once, I wish I could hear those words. Friends send cards and come to see her. They seem to forget that I even exist. There are days I feel worthless!"

Because of the intense demands on caregivers, there is little time for them to be refreshed through personal pursuits or to take care of themselves. Through their own eyes they may appear worthless. However, looking at themselves through Christ's grace-filled eyes offers them a view of their worth beyond all comprehension!

Caregiver, your Creator knows the number of hairs left in your comb today and the number left on your head! An average heart pumps between 1,500 to 2,000 gallons of blood daily, but God knows exactly how much blood your heart pumped today and even the amount of blood you lose from a tiny scratch!

God loved what He made with His hands so much that He took on human flesh in a womb so He could suffer and die to redeem us. Jesus did not die for sparrows. He died for you! Never doubt your worth! Caregiver, your worth is not in what you *do* but in who you are: God's redeemed child!

God's child—priceless!

4 Trust

Trust Him with the Missing Pieces

Delight yourself in the LORD, . . . Commit your way to the LORD; trust in Him. Psalm 37:4–5

I am so glad Jesus is my caregiver. The pain and suffering of the past two decades have been the catalysts that helped me to mature emotionally, mentally, and spiritually. I feel confident and independent, trusting in the Lord for my physical and emotional needs. The challenges that were set before me were overwhelming, and at times I thought I wouldn't make it out of the quagmire that was pulling me down.

First, my husband went through several years of clinical depression until doctors found the right medication. Next, my mom developed Alzheimer's, and it saddened me that I could no longer have those lovely mother-daughter chats. My widowed out-of-state aunt had no children to care for her affairs and chose to stay independent; she gave power of attorney to her lawyer's secretary. The HIPPA Act created problems in that her nearest relatives—my brother and I—had no rights to be contacted on her behalf. A few years later, my stepmother developed lung cancer. That set us on a collision course with an unscrupulous caregiver who seemed to take over my dad's life following my stepmother's death. That was almost my undoing!

Five different situations, but not one is unique to just me. Caregivers around the world face these same situations and more on a daily basis. But we get through our challenges because we trust in God. Life is a puzzle where many of the pieces don't fit. We need to turn them right-side-up to see the pattern and turn them slowly to see the connection to other puzzle pieces. Some pieces may be missing. Perhaps God wants us to put as much of the puzzle together as we can, then trust Him with the missing pieces.

Jesus tells us, "I am the way, and the truth, and the life" (John 14:6). He remains steadfast. He alone reconciles us to the Father. He fulfills all of our needs, rescuing us from our sin, and slipping perfectly fitting pieces into place. Jesus is our caregiver. He loves us, delights in being with us, has compassion for us and, most important, shows us the way to eternal life with the Father.

Trust Him with your life's puzzle pieces!

5 Respite
Do You Need a Break Today?

And He said to them, "Come away by yourselves to a desolate place and rest a while." For many were coming and going, and they had no leisure even to eat. Mark 6:31

1. Which sentence describes you?

> I am a caregiver.
>
> I am not a caregiver.

Most people have been a caregiver, will become one, or are one right now. There are approximately sixty-five million caregivers in the United States today. You are not alone.

2. Which sentence describes you as a caregiver?

> I am exhausted.
>
> I am refreshed.
>
> I have nothing to do.

Each day can be physically demanding and mentally overwhelming. Whether you are a hands-on or long-distance caregiver, whether your loved one lives with you or in a special care facility, caregiving is a treadmill life that just keeps going with no time to stop and get off. Would you agree?

3. Have you ever needed a respite?

       Yes.

       No.

Respite is defined as a temporary rest or relief. Caregivers don't think they need a break. Some ask, "What would people think if I asked for help?"

Plain and simple, if you do not take care of yourself, you will not be able to take care of your loved one. This is not a sign of inadequacy but of being smart when you ask for help. Whether you take a five-minute walk or an hour-long trip to the grocery store, even a short break will help you re-fresh. Respites are energy boosters both physically and mentally!

Daily sitting at the feet of your Savior, who gave His life that you may have abundant life, is where real respite happens. In these be-still-and-know-that-I-am-God moments of respite, we become a portable sanctuary. Here we find hope and contentment, wisdom and boldness to do what is right even when it hurts. Time with Jesus is not running from the world, it is running to your Savior, who will restore your body and soul!

Jesus' disciples were caregivers comforting

others also. Jesus knew His disciples needed a break. He knows this about you too. Listen to His voice: "Come with Me by yourselves to a quiet place and get some rest" (Mark 6:31 NIV). Will you?

4. What kind of respite will you begin today?

> Make the five minutes you take for a
>   cup of coffee a time of prayer.
> Before getting out of bed, read a
>   few verses of Scripture.
> Keep a book of devotions in the car to
>   read while waiting at appointments.
> *Be refreshed in His presence!*

6 Time for God's Word
Are You Thirsty?

Your word is a lamp to my feet and a light to my path.
Psalm 119:105

I am so limited in time to sit down and read God's Word. My caregiving is taking more of my time. I am so thirsty for words of comfort. When will I find a few minutes to sit and quench my thirst, be refilled and refueled so I can keep going? I know that it takes only a short time being in God's Word to feel His Spirit strengthening my tired, exhausted body, but it's getting more difficult to snatch even a few minutes to read the Bible.

Whether or not I can find those few minutes to sit down and read my Bible, I can recall my Baptism, as well as the words and verses I learned from my Sunday School teachers and others who have helped plant the seeds of God's love in me. I think of Timothy and his mother, Eunice, as she daily passed her faith in the Gospel along to him. Lois, his grandmother, did the same. I imagine the wonderful stories of Jesus they shared with Timothy that created in him a strong faith in those Gospel promises. May God bless those seeds of love that always quench my thirst, for they enable His love and faithfulness to bloom in my heart for the challenges to come.

God's Word lights my path!

7 Patience
Rocky Soil of Life

Other seeds fell on rocky ground, where they did not have much soil, and immediately they sprang up, since they had no depth of soil. Matthew 13:5

As I sat waiting for the test results, I couldn't help but notice outside my window the beautiful trees emerging from their winter hibernation. They were covered with gorgeous pink blooms, and yet they were growing in rocky soil. That's the way I feel today. I'm in the rocky soil of life. I feel like my legs are too heavy to move—like rocks weighing down heavily on plant roots. I seem to get tired so easily these days. I'm impatient, short with others, and frustrated when things don't happen in *my* time.

Although I'm weighed down, I think of what Jesus did for me when He died and rose again, and I feel connected and balanced once more. Jesus is my source for living. I am a branch connected to Him through Baptism. He enables me to bloom with a smile and helps me find ways to see positive outcomes to negative situations, such as my impatience, that could overwhelm me.

Caregivers provide for their loved ones twenty-four hours a day, seven days a week. What a joy it is to be assured that God's love is there for me as I minister to my loved one. Keeping myself rooted in Christ and watered by His Word will strengthen me by the grace that is in Christ Jesus to continue to provide care and love and to "bear fruit with patience" (Luke 8:15).

The living Word—my source!

8 Sleep
Sleep Will Come

I will lie down and sleep in peace, for You alone, O Lord, make me dwell in safety. Psalm 4:8 NIV

Sleep doesn't come easily for caregivers. You feel like you don't want to be too far away from your loved one because you're afraid you won't hear a call for help. You might feel that if you stay awake, it will help the situation. But is that really true?

David, the psalmist, could have had sleepless nights when his son Absalom rebelled and gathered an army to kill him. But he slept peacefully, even during the rebellion. What made the difference? David cried out to the Lord, and the Lord heard him. The assurance of answered prayers brings peace. It's easier to sleep well when we have full assurance that God is in control of circumstances. Whether you lie awake with concerns or get a good night's sleep, what joy it is to know we have full assurance that God is in control of every situation.

Jesus had no trouble sleeping. While He and His disciples were in a boat on the sea, a storm arose with great winds that threatened to swamp the boat. The disciples were frightened, but Jesus slept on. When they awakened Him, He calmed the winds and waves, and the disciples marveled at the kind of man He was that even the winds and waves obeyed Him (Matthew 8:23–27).

If you are lying awake at night, worrying about situations you can't change, pour out your heart to God, and thank Him that He is in control. Then rest in the peace that only He can give.

God is in control!

9 Impatience
I Want Answers Now!

Answer me when I call to You, O my righteous God.
Give me relief from my distress; be merciful to me
and hear my prayer. Psalm 4:1 NIV

Have you ever questioned God's timing in answering your prayers? We all have. But when the stress of caregiving looms before you, it becomes even more urgent to have your questions answered *now*. It's difficult to wait.

King David knew that God would hear him when he called and would answer. We, too, can be confident that God listens to our prayers and answers when we call on Him. If we trust Christ for our salvation, God will listen to us and answer. "For I know the plans I have for you, declares the LORD, plans for welfare and not for evil, to give you a future and a hope" (Jeremiah 29:11).

When you feel as though your prayers are bouncing off the ceiling, remember that as a believer, you have been set apart by God and that He loves you. He hears and answers your prayers, although His answers may not be what you expect.

Look at your problems in the light of God's power instead of looking at God in the shadow of your problems. "But I trust in You, O LORD; I say, 'You are my God.' My times are in Your hand" (Psalm 31:14–15).

God's timing is perfect!

10 Joy of the Cross
The Real Joy in Our Journey

For the joy of the LORD is your strength. Nehemiah 8:10

There is a story of a young man who was at the end of his rope. Seeing no way out, he dropped to his knees in prayer. "Lord, I can't go on," he said. "I have too heavy a cross to bear."

The Lord replied, "My son, if you can't bear its weight, just place your cross inside this room. Then, open that other door and pick out any cross you wish."

The man was filled with relief and said, "Thank You, Lord," and he did as he was told.

Upon entering the other room, he saw many crosses, some so large that the tops were not visible.

Then, he spotted a tiny cross leaning against a far wall. "I'd like that one, Lord," he whispered.

The Lord replied, "My son, that is the cross you just brought in."

Although each caregiver's situation is different, we still have one thing in common: our burdens are heavy! Jesus, our caregiver, personally understands what we are going through. Because of the joy set before Him, He endured the cross so that we will not grow weary and lose heart. His joy is our strength.

The real joy we have through Jesus Christ is quite different from happiness. Happiness is external and temporary because it depends upon circumstances, which continually change. Real joy is internal and permanent because we trust God who never changes! Real joy is rooted in the death of Jesus Christ on the cross, and our new life began when He walked out of the tomb and ascended into heaven! That gives us security and strength for every single detail in our caregiving journey. Nothing can ever take His joy from us!

His presence is the joy in our journey!

11 Trying to Do It All
No Problem . . . Help!!

I can do all things through Him who strengthens me.
Philippians 4:13

No problem. I can handle this! were my thoughts the first time someone referred to me as the caregiver for my dad. All I have to do is call more often, do his laundry once a week, and make a few extra casseroles. No big deal!

As the weeks went by, my own daily routine was no longer the norm. I had to face reality. The care receiver's needs are all-consuming twenty-four hours a day, seven days a week. I was exhausted, stressed out, and snapping like a rubber band at my family, co-workers, and even my failing dad.

I fell to my knees and pleaded with God to forgive me for thinking that *I* could handle this new role in life by myself! God already knew what I now shamefully admitted. I prayed, but forgot to give the day back to Him. I called on His help only when I was desperate. *I* could handle everything. Oh, how Satan loved to blur my vision from the grace of God and His everlasting strength.

Satan loves it when I think that life looks impossible. And it does—until I remember that I live in God's grace. It is by Christ's sacrifice on the cross that I can be forgiven and know that I am His redeemed child.

From that day on, I began a new routine before I even got out of bed in the morning. I praised God for blessing me with a new day to show His love through me to my dad, no matter how challenging that might be. Then I reaffirmed to God that *I* can do nothing without Him but that I can do everything *through* Him who gives me strength.

Walk with the Savior!

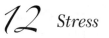 **Stress**

Stress Is Good?

Then they cried to the LORD in their trouble,
and He delivered them from their distress. . . .
For He satisfies the longing soul, and the hungry soul
He fills with good things. Psalm 107:6, 9

If I have learned only one thing from caregiving, it is this: there is a lot of stress! I've read that whenever there is change, stress becomes attached to it. In caregiving there are many changes. Your loved one is no longer the same, whether the change is physical or behavioral. As you care for your loved one, the changes affect your family, friends, and even your church family because you yourself are changing. You're sometimes tired, grumpy, and worried, and these attributes begin to become part of your daily attitude.

"Who of you by worrying can add a single hour to his life? Since you cannot do this very little thing, why do you worry about the rest?" (Luke 12:25–26 NIV). God uses the stresses of life for His good purpose. Stress was laced throughout the lives of Paul and Silas. For instance, Paul and Silas were wrongfully beaten and imprisoned, yet they were content to stay where they were when an earthquake opened their prison doors. They used this opportunity to share with the jailer the Good News that those who believe in Jesus as their Savior shall not perish but have eternal life.

The joy of the Gospel will always take the sting out of stress even on a caregiver's worst day. What a joy to share with our loved ones that we only have to believe in Jesus as our Savior and trust in Him!

His steadfast love endures forever!

13 Hope
God's Little Surprises

Rejoice in hope, be patient in tribulation, be constant in prayer. Romans 12:12

The mail today arrived with bills, bills, and more bills, or so I thought. I immediately felt devastated to have to open so many heartaches. I looked at the addresses. Yes, we had been to those places for tests. How could anything else be inside that envelope but another bill!

However, today was different. The insurance paid more than I had anticipated. Several turned out to be those "This Is Not a Bill" statements. I love those! What a relief! I love God's little surprises in my life today.

Right now I have no clue how we'll be able to pay our mounting bills, but I know that just as God provided these surprises today for me, I have hope. He is a God of details. He knows exactly what I need even when I don't. Look how He cared for all mankind by sending His Son to walk among us and feel the hurts and stresses that we feel. Then He allowed His Son to die on the cross so that all who believe in Him will have redemption by His blood. His resurrection points us toward eternal life with Him. That's a *huge* God-surprise for all of us!

I can hope because God is my caregiver. I can already feel an inner peace. I'm glad God and I are in this caregiving business together.

God is my caregiver!

14 Carrying It Alone
Carry It Alone? No Way!

Sing for joy to God our strength; shout aloud to the God of Jacob! . . . He says, "I removed the burden from their shoulders; their hands were set free."
Psalm 81:1, 6

Certainly that can't be true, I thought, but the scales do not lie. I wasn't surprised though. Eating seems to relieve the continual challenges of a caregiver. Food offers comfort. The problem was that eating is only temporary, so I continued to worry and eat and worry and eat.

It never ceases to amaze me how God works to offer His comfort. My parents had always read the Bible together, then left it lying open on the kitchen table. One day I glanced at the verse on the top of the page. It was like God used His heavenly highlighter and circled it just for me.

"Take My yoke upon you and learn from Me. . . . For My yoke is easy and My burden is light" (Matthew 11:29–30). I had always thought that yoking animals together was cruel and awkward. However, in truth, the yoke is a blessing because it enables them to share their burdens and to walk in unity.

That describes the caregiver's relationship to Jesus. Rather than being yoked to our burdens, we are joined with the love and strength of our Baptism and the forgiveness of sins. Caregivers often view themselves as heavily yoked to the care receiver; however, they should feel themselves joyfully yoked to Jesus. How thankful we are that our Lord Jesus stepped into our place to accept our sins on our behalf. Through this unselfish act, God gives us the free gift of eternal life with Him.

Trusting in God's tailor-made plan for us truly lightens our load and may even help us feel pounds lighter.

Yoked to God is a blessing!

15 *Living Stones*
You Are Living Stones

As you come to Him, the living Stone—
rejected by men but chosen by God and precious
to Him—you also, like living stones, are being built
into a spiritual house to be a holy priesthood,
offering spiritual sacrifices acceptable to God
through Jesus Christ. 1 Peter 2:4–5 NIV

Sometimes caregivers are angry and frustrated with the many responsibilities they have, and occasionally they resent the assumption that they alone will take on the role of caregiver. While other family members go about their normal daily schedule, you must squeeze your schedule within the parameters of another's needs.

Peter offers an interesting perspective to our function and worth in God's kingdom. He refers to us as "living stones" in God's spiritual house. Each person, like each stone of a temple, is carefully chosen and placed to bring strength and beauty to the structure. A temple cannot be made with only one stone. Keeping this in mind, we can feel confident and justified when we share caregiving responsibilities with family members, friends, and professionals.

Peter goes on to remind us that we are a holy priesthood, bringing spiritual sacrifices that are highly valued by God. He looks with favor on acts of worship, praise, good works, the sacrifice of possessions, and the time we give in service. These, too, are common sacrifices that go along with the role of caregiving. God loves our selfless service, which is built on the Cornerstone, Jesus Christ, who shed His blood to make us righteous before God.

Living stones centered on Christ!

16 Decisions
What Am I to Do?

Jesus' disciples asked Him, "Where do You want us to go and make preparations for You to eat the Passover?" . . . [Jesus said,] "Go into the city, and a man carrying a jar of water will meet you. Follow him." Mark 14:12–13

There came a time when my mother could no longer manage living in her own home. Alzheimer's disease was robbing her of her judgment, and she needed round-the-clock supervision. Throughout her life, she had made my brother and me promise never to put her in a nursing home, but at that time we never dreamt that mom would have mental lapses and make decisions to run away from home in the middle of the night wearing only her night-gown and slippers. It became apparent that she needed a professional facility that could keep her safe and take care of her special needs.

The disciples faced a different challenge for making arrangements for the Passover Feast. Jesus gave a detailed answer to their question. How I longed for Jesus to give me the same detailed an-swer to my question, "Oh, God, what am I to do?" I can look back now and see that the Lord did lead me and even prepared the way.

Mom didn't like her new assisted living home for many months. I learned to accept the circum-stances and continued to trust in my heavenly Fa-ther to guide the decisions that had to be made over the next few years.

The decisions that the disciples made are in-spiring. We are told that when Jesus asked them to follow Him, they left their families, their careers, and all they had. Did they know what lay ahead for them? Did they know they were following the true Son of God? Did they know they were following the Messiah, the Savior? What may have started

as an adventure—following the Master Teacher—
ended in a revolution that changed the world.

Decision-making for the care of our parents
is accompanied by fear and sometimes sadness.
The roles of parent and child have been reversed,
and we feel totally out of our element. Yet we are
not alone; there is hope. The Lord delights in being part of our decision making and continues to be
right beside us, preparing the way.

Jesus, my guide and my strength!

17 Disabled Child
Hope for the Journey

*Be strong and courageous. Do not fear or be in dread …
for it is the LORD your God who goes with you.
He will not leave you or forsake you.* Deuteronomy 31:6

"I'm sorry to tell you this, but the news is not
good. Your child has ____." My heart sank to the
deepest depth of the ocean after the doctor's diagnosis. It doesn't matter whether the diagnosis is cancer,
Duchenne Muscular Dystrophy, Down syndrome,
or another disease that strikes fear in a parent's

heart and changes her lifestyle forever. The feelings are the same. Cheering at soccer games was our plan, not coaching our child through the next stage of the disease.

The initial diagnosis leaves the parents in a fog, not knowing what to do next except follow the outline on the doctor's paper regarding where they need to be and when. Trying to make sense of terminology that is totally foreign—chemotherapy, radiation, braces, wheelchair—is incredibly difficult. These are for *my* child? My sweet, adorable child who has barely been touched by the world yet?

To caregivers, knowledge is key to caring for a loved one. Learn all you can from the Internet, libraries, blogs, and support groups. Groups, whether in your town or online, can give you much-needed encouragement and hope.

You are never alone! Be assured that this journey will be hope-filled because God is holding your hand and walking this walk with you. That is security for the known and the unknown! He understands the anxiety of your aching heart. He knows exactly how many tears you shed, and that is okay. Jesus wept too. Never underestimate, though, the unique ways He will continually interlace His grace and mercy throughout your day. Trust in His faithfulness with all your heart and strength.

He passionately loves you. To prove this, God sacrificed His Son Jesus on a cross. Certainly He could have called on thousands of angels to save Him, but He didn't. Belief in Jesus' death and resurrection gives us eternal life. That's *guaranteed hope* for you and your child!

God's love—our hope!

18 *Self-Care*
Who, Me? Exercise?

But those who hope in the LORD will renew their strength. They will soar on wings like eagles; they will run and not grow weary, they will walk and not be faint. Isaiah 40:31 NIV

"A caregiver does not have time to think about her racing heart, back pain, or blood pressure when there is a wheelchair to be lifted in and out of the car or the next dialysis appointment to keep," thought Patty after being rushed to the emergency room.

Caregivers do an admirable job of taking care of their loved ones but typically compromise their own health. Self-care is as important as oxygen.

Without it, you could have a shorter lifespan than you expect, and you wouldn't be able to help others effectively.

While many caregivers report feeling loved, appreciated, and needed, there are still complex responsibilities and demands on their time, energy, and finances. Stress expresses itself through increased irritability, forgetfulness, loss of energy or zest for life, and even loss of a sense of humor.

"If I couldn't laugh at myself, I would be crying all the time," laughed a caregiver. "We who give care need to laugh and play in order to balance out our heavy burdens. It's a measure of sound mental health to be able to look squarely at the frustrations that plague us, even if there is nothing to laugh about. Laugh because it is good for your health!"

Patty was given a list of wellness tips in the ER. "I can't do this. My time is not really *my* time," she said. The doctor nodded, but added, "We've found that the major reason caregivers won't even go for a five-minute walk or do some stretching exercises while sitting with their loved one is the lack of support and encouragement to do so." Then he asked, "Patty, who will you ask to be your support team, and when will you ask them?"

On the drive home, Patty cried as she talked with God about her stress. She then asked for guidance and mercy. She committed herself to daily exercise beginning first in her walk with the Lord and keeping her Bible *out* on the table and *open* where she could inhale hope throughout the day. Jesus and His disciples walked everywhere. Our Lord even walked the rugged path to the cross on Golgotha so we can be His redeemed children.

Strength Warm-Up

> *Stretch* up to God.
> *Reach* out and be His hands.
> *Bow* down in respect.
> *Kick* sin away.
> *Jump* for JOY and praise God!

> —Diana Schnack

19 Loneliness
Where Did My Friends Go?

Turn to me and be gracious to me, for I am lonely and afflicted. Psalm 25:16

"Some people come into our lives and quickly go. Some stay for a while and leave footprints on our hearts. And we are never the same." —Author Unknown

During my caregiving years, I began to notice my friends didn't stop by as much, and after a while they didn't call as often either. What had changed? I was still the same person—or was I?

Being a caregiver is challenging. The demands on your time can leave you so tired that you lose your ability to think clearly. Forgetfulness is a big part of your day for things other than the needs of your loved one. But you need that support from your friends to keep you focused. What can you do?

First, if you notice your friends not calling as often, it could be because they don't want to interrupt your caregiving duties. Let them know that you want them to leave a message, and you'll return their call. Tell them how much you need their support. Ask them not to quit calling or stopping by. Friendship is like a little piece of charcoal. When lit and separated from the others, it will soon extinguish itself. However, once placed back with the other bits of embers, it soon starts burning again. In the same way, we all need friends to keep us going. Their encouragement is critical.

Jesus was always an encourager to His friends Mary, Martha, and Lazarus. This was evidenced four days after the death of Lazarus when Jesus arrived, and both Mary and Martha said to Him,

"Lord, if You had been here, my brother would not have died" (John 11:21). Look at the faith these women had even in their grief! Jesus did raise Lazarus from the dead; Mary and Martha and others saw the Son of God at work in their midst.

What a friend we have in Jesus! With Jesus as your friend, you'll be able to keep your light burning for your friends and all to see.

Radiate God's love!

20 Depression
Hope in All Things

For we were so utterly burdened beyond our strength that we despaired of life itself.
Indeed, we felt that we had received the sentence of death. But that was to make us rely not on ourselves but on God who raises the dead.

2 Corinthians 1:8b–9

Taking care of someone else can be challenging. Taking care of yourself in the process is often more difficult. No matter how much you love or think of the person you look after, it is no wonder that you can feel low at times.

It is important that you get as much help and support as possible. That can be long- or short-term support in the form of seeking respite care, employing support caregivers, involving family or friends more, finding residential care for your loved one, or enlisting help to give you more time for yourself. Local support groups are fantastic.

Depression is emotional heaviness that weighs down the heart. The apostle Paul used the Greek word *bareo* which means "pressed or weighed down" to describe the immense emotional pressure that he and Timothy suffered at the hands of those who opposed Christ (2 Corinthians 1:8-9).

In Psalm 6, David writes of six symptoms of depression: faintness of heart, agony of body, anguish of soul, weariness from groaning, a pillow stained with tears, and eyes weak from sorrow. Psalm 102 demonstrates that the righteous can get depressed. The psalmist describes his loss of appetite, sleeplessness, constant weeping, and darkness.

Being together with God in prayer can be beneficial when you're downhearted. It brings you closer to your heavenly Father. Jesus gave His life so we have hope when all seems hopeless. In Psalm 42, the psalmist advises us to put our hope in God and to do it by praising Him.

May the God of hope fill you with all joy
and peace as you trust in Him, so that
you may overflow with hope by the
power of the Holy Spirit. Romans 15:13 NIV

Hope in His unfailing love!

21 *Guilt*
A Bag of Burdens

*Out of my distress I called on the LORD; the LORD
answered me and set me free.* Psalm 118:5

A caregiver is like the elderly man who was
walking along the road, bent over from carrying a
heavy backpack. A tractor pulling a wagon stopped,
and the driver offered him a ride. He joyfully accepted. But when seated, he kept holding his heavy
load. "Why don't you lay down your burden?" asked
the driver. The man replied, "I feel that it is almost
too much to ask you to carry me, and I couldn't
think of letting you carry my burdens too."

For a caregiver, this heavy burden is often
guilt.

- "If only I made her go to the doctor sooner."

- "I promised I would always take care of her at home."

- "I feel so guilty for raising my voice and upsetting her."

- "What will people think if I go out with my friends?"

Caregiving is a very intensive and emotional season. Numerous thoughts and feelings well up, and they are not totally controllable, even when we are at our best; much less so under the strain of giving care. Lamenting over our feelings of guilt does not mean we love anyone less. It is a human response!

Draw strength from the Psalms. From deep distress to glorious joy-filled praise, David expressed himself as he called on the Lord. God accepts us just as He did the psalmists.

Jesus gave His life so we can lay our burdens at the foot of His cross. His resurrection has set us free from our guilt and proved His passionate love for us because He personally wants to carry each burden we have! That's real joy!

Freed through His resurrection!

22 Listening
Are You Listening?

And He said, "He who has ears to hear, let him hear."
Mark 4:9

"You hear, but why don't you listen?" my mother used to ask me. Do you listen when you hear others talk?

Psychologists say one of the greatest things we can do for another is to listen. No interruptions. No walking away, reading the paper, watching TV. Listening is a priceless gift.

Respect is a key to becoming a good listener. And not just listening, but also hearing the emotions and conflict beneath spoken words. That's true loyalty.

Many times caregivers hear their loved one repeating the same things over and over and over. We tune them out and turn them off. Guilty! But be assured you are not alone. It would be difficult to find someone who hasn't appeared to be listening to another while her mind is making a grocery list.

People who are suffering frequently want to talk about their situation and feelings—if we let them. Good questions can open gushers, and then healing begins, in part because you as the caregiver are gaining information to help the person, but mostly because he or she is talking and you are listening. Never underestimate the profound power of listening.

A quick glance at the Psalms shows that those who wrote them often pleaded with God to listen and wondered why He seemed so far away in their times of trouble. As a caregiver, can you relate to questioning God through your tears? The psalmists did. Psalm 22 shows us the progression from wondering if God is listening to calming down and realizing that we can trust that He listens. Whatever Psalm you read, you will find comfort.

We can pour out endless praises to God for listening and showing us how valuable we are to Him. Jesus Christ was beaten and nailed to a cross, but it didn't end there. Three days later He was alive! Listen to those eternal life-giving words: He is *alive*! For Jesus' sake, isn't this all the more reason we should really stop and listen to the words of our loved ones?

Listen with your heart!

23 *Family Conflict*
Family Stress and Conflict

Starting a quarrel is like breaching a dam; so drop the matter before a dispute breaks out. Proverbs 17:14 NIV

When a loved one is diagnosed with a debilitating disease such as dementia, multiple sclerosis, cancer, and the like, the effects on your family can be overwhelming. The reality that someone you love has such a devastating illness can trigger a range of emotions including fear, sadness, confusion, and anger. Conflicts are common as family members struggle with the new paradigm of dealing with the situation. Working through conflicts together, though, can help you and your family move on to more important things—namely, caring for your loved one and enjoying your time together as much as possible. Deal with difficult emotions right away. Don't sacrifice the relationship for the situation.

Jacob's family life had been a long, broken record of deceit and rivalry. Jacob cheats Esau, Laban cheats Jacob, Laban exploits Jacob, Jacob flees, Laban chases Jacob, and on and on. Through it all, there is a thread weaving in and out that shows

God's mighty hand at work. Eventually Jacob and Laban realize their destructive behavior is hurting the entire family and their relationship with God. They stop, share a meal, and make a covenant with God to not harm each other again (Genesis 31).

Our sins, which enslave us, were drowned when we were baptized into Jesus' death and resurrection. In the Word of God, we look into our loving Creator's eyes and see His mercy toward us in Christ Jesus. Family conflict falls away, and we, like all believers, have a new start in Him.

God's mercies are new each morning!

24 Attitudes
Equipped for the Challenge

But [Jesus] said to me, "My grace is sufficient for you, for My power is made perfect in weakness." Therefore I will boast all the more gladly of my weaknesses, so that the power of Christ may rest upon me. 2 Corinthians 12:9

When I first became a caregiver, I pleaded with God that He had the wrong person. I didn't know anything about caring for a disabled person. Sticking to a routine was not for me and neither was staying home. I was impatient if I had to sit and wait at appointments because I liked to be in control! *No, God, I am not equipped to be a patient, calm caregiver.*

The reality is that God not only uses flawed vessels, it is His plan and delight to do so. Abraham was old. Moses stuttered. Gideon was afraid. The disciples fell asleep while praying. Naomi had a bad attitude. Martha worried!

God asks us to remember whenever we doubt our abilities that He will never ask us to do anything for which He has not first equipped us. We can *trust* Him on that! We can step out, fully confident, knowing that He will make us capable. He is faithful to His promises!

St. Paul tells us that our problems and weaknesses show our need for God. With no burdens or problems, we would have no need for a Savior. Through our caregiving challenges we remember the pain and suffering Jesus Christ endured to give us access to the Father and to heaven. We rely on His grace and mercy to lift us up. His presence equips us as we walk through our caregiving season.

God's grace—always sufficient!

25 Attitudes
How's Your Attitude?

Rejoice in the Lord always; . . . do not be anxious
about anything, but in everything by prayer
and supplication with thanksgiving let your requests
be made known to God. And the peace of God,
which surpasses all understanding, will guard
your hearts and your minds in Christ Jesus.
Philippians 4:4, 6–7

There was once a useless mule that fell into an old well. Its owner, a farmer, decided that since he used neither the well nor the mule anymore he would fill the well with dirt and bury the mule while he was at it. As the farmer shoved dirt into the well, the mule kept feeling it hit him on his back. Whenever he felt dirt hit him, he shook it off onto the ground. As the dirt filled the well, the mule took a step up. Shovelful after shovelful, the mule shook off the dirt and stepped up. Eventually there was enough dirt in the well that the mule was able to simply step out of it. What an attitude!

One challenge most caregivers would love to shake off is the inability to control the dynamics of their day. As a caregiver, you have no control over an agency's unreturned telephone call, physicians who take vacations when you need them most, or your loved one's need for help when you are exhausted. However, you do have a choice about your attitude. You can either take your bad attitude out on those around you or *rejoice* because you *trust* that Jesus Christ is, has been, and always will be in control of all things. He proved this when the sadness of Good Friday was followed with Easter morning jubilation!

Even through shipwrecks and beatings, Paul learned that a rejoicing attitude always flows from a heart rooted in Christ. He teaches us that our internal attitudes do not have to reflect our external circumstances. The key to contentment and thanksgiving is to draw on the saving grace of Jesus Christ and His strength through His Holy Word, prayer, and supplication. Do not base your life on circumstances, but on God's grace. That revives our attitude!

Rejoice in the Lord always!

26 *Prodigal Caregiver*

The Prodigal Caregiver

Forgive us our debts, as we also have forgiven our debtors. Matthew 6:12

"Thank You, Jesus, for letting me be a caregiver!"

Wait. Did I really say that? Absolutely, and from a grateful heart overflowing with God's grace and forgiveness.

I grew up with a mother who made sure I was baptized and attended Sunday School and church every Sunday, and vacation Bible school every summer. My siblings and I even had to listen to her read the Bible almost daily. As the years passed, though, I began to think, *This is not for me! Why do I need this?*

When it came time for the teen youth group, I was at the age when I thought I knew everything. I left home; I wanted to travel far away. Enough of this Jesus stuff. I headed for greener pastures. But that old cliché—the grass is always greener on the other side of the road—just isn't true. I got in with the wrong group of kids, did things I never should have done, and ended up living under a bridge with other homeless people.

There was a kind lady who came to us with hot chocolate early in the mornings. She reminded me so much of my mother, and I longed to return home. I hadn't kept in contact with her directly, but I knew what was happening there. I heard she'd had a stroke and wasn't doing too well. I wanted to go back, but could I apologize and ask for forgiveness after all the heartbreak I had caused her? The more I thought about it, what did I have to lose?

Today as I sit by her bedside, I am praising God that He put all the pieces in place for me to re-enter the lives of my family. As I look at my mother, she can only make a lopsided smile and gently squeeze my hand, but that's enough for me.

I am grateful for this caregiving time. It gives me a chance to show her how sorry I am for hurting her. But more important, I want God to know how grateful I am for His grace and forgiveness. It's amazing how much of what I listened to when I was younger comes back to me. I have learned that to forgive is not excusing or forgetting the wrong. The benefit of remembering is that it encourages gratitude, extinguishes pride, and exhibits grace. "A man's wisdom gives him patience; it is his glory to overlook an offense" (Proverbs 19:11 NIV).

By the grace of God, Jesus' suffering for our sins became a passport to our wholeness and everlasting joy. Through His death and resurrection, our hurting hearts are healed. My mother taught me that if I believe that Jesus Christ died and rose again, I never have to doubt my eternal life. Thanks, Mom. I love you!

Forgiveness—real joy!

27 Special Occasions Celebrate Life!

Be joyful at your Feast. Deuteronomy 16:14

"Tommy, your grandma and grandpa won't be able to come to your birthday celebration this year," said mom as she was setting the table and placing candy favors at each place setting.

"What do you mean? We can't have my birthday dinner without Grandma and Grandpa!" exclaimed eight-year-old Tommy.

"Well, Grandma is just not able to get out of bed anymore, Honey. Grandpa needs to stay by her side right now. But we can celebrate your special day with Uncle Josh and Aunt Grace. That will be nice, won't it?"

"Yeah, I guess," Tommy sighed dejectedly as he stared at the floor. "It just won't be the same."

"I know, Sweetie. I agree with you that it won't be the same, but sometimes as we're growing up, things change. It's part of life. You know what? After everybody leaves, let's take some cake over to Grandma and Grandpa. There are many different ways to celebrate. Just remember that shut-ins like to participate, too, only in their own way."

"Yeah! I like that idea!" yelled Tommy.

Precious caregiver, when we find ourselves in times of stress and hardship, our inclination is to skip the celebrations. But God wants His people to take time to celebrate life and to enjoy fellowship together. His instructions for the people included feasts and festivals—a chance to break from work, to rejoice, to sing, to dance, and to give Him thanks.

Sometimes our reluctance to celebrate is understandable and legitimate; however, it does not take away our respect and concern for our loved one. But such occasions can be God-given opportunities to find relief from the day-to-day struggle of staying afloat spiritually, emotionally, and physically. They are times to refocus on His gifts: friends, family, food, music. And even small celebrations—

a quiet family dinner, a stop for ice cream, a walk through the local park, or even just a break for a cup of tea with a friend—can give us a renewed awareness that God is so good.

God's gift to us to celebrate is His Son. He gave Himself to us in the person of Jesus Christ who humbled Himself to become flesh to walk among us. He then laid down His life as He took our sins upon Himself, but the Good News to celebrate is His resurrection. After He rose from the dead, He walked among His disciples and friends for forty days before ascending into heaven. Wow! That is something to celebrate!

Celebrate His victory over death!

28 Long-Distance Caregiving
Holding Hands with Jesus

I am the LORD; I have called you in righteousness;
I will take you by the hand and keep you. Isaiah 42:6

True or false? Long-distance caregivers have much less stress than those who live close to their care receiver.

False. Long-distance caregivers experience many of the same feelings of guilt and depression as nearby caregivers. However, the geographical distance can make the situation more complicated. If you are a long-distance caregiver, you may not feel as fatigued as the hands-on caregiver, but living farther away does not make you immune to feeling worried and anxious.

Long-distance caregiving takes an enormous amount of physical and psychological energy. You can't go immediately when the care receiver needs you, assess his or her well-being firsthand, or feel like you are doing enough. While with your loved one, time flies away as you take time to verify his or her checkbook, change light bulbs, check the noise in the car, restock the refrigerator, and get an update from the neighbors (along with some criticism because you live so far away). All the while you try to remain calm because your loved one wants you to sit down and listen to him or her talk. Caregiving can bring on a full range of human emotions. Is it any wonder you are so hard on yourself? Don't give up, though; there is hope!

Accept the fact that although *you* cannot always be present, *God* is!

Affirm for yourself the types of care you can provide from far away for both your loved one and the primary caregiver. Pray for the Holy Spirit's guidance to use you to be an encourager and to provide emotional support as a listener through phone calls. Remind your care receiver of your love but focus on God's everlasting love!

Assure your loved one that whether you are together or separated by distance, you are each God's forgiven and redeemed child through the death and resurrection of His Son, Jesus Christ. Rejoice together that as you navigate your way through these caregiving situations, everything is in God's hands.

Hand-in-hand with Jesus = security!

29 Making a Difference
Candid Camera Caregivers

*But you are a chosen race, a royal priesthood,
a holy nation, a people for His own possession,
that you may proclaim the excellencies of Him who
called you out of darkness into His marvelous light.*
1 Peter 2:9

"You're a candid camera caregiver!" Edie told

her friend Julia. "I've watched you for many years, and as a caregiver you witness more than you will ever realize."

Julia laughed. "That's the first time I've heard a caregiver described like that. I don't think of myself as a witness. I just take care of Mom. Although some days can be very challenging, I still try to take her places with me. At times I'm a little embarrassed at the way she does and says things at the grocery store or in a restaurant. But now that I understand that this is all part of the aging process, I'm a lot less stressed. I just let people think whatever they want. I know Mom has a good heart."

Edie interrupted, "That is exactly what I mean about being on candid camera. When you least expect that anyone is watching, others see you naturally fulfilling the caregiver's role and how you react and respond to various situations. You are making a difference by helping others see the caregiving season with a new perspective!"

Precious caregiver, just as the Good Samaritan showed mercy and made a difference in the disabled man's life, Jesus instructs us to "go, and do likewise" (Luke 10:37). Making a difference is nothing we do on our own! It is Christ working in and through us as we glorify Him. Transformation in our attitude and actions began at our Baptism and continues as we spend time in His Word and in prayer.

Christ's death and resurrection make an eternal difference in our lives! Because of that hope, we can walk boldly through the caregiving season witnessing His love through our individual uniqueness!

Smile! You are a picture of Christ today!

30 Psalm 23
My Shepherd, My Caregiver

The LORD is my shepherd.

Because I am your shepherd and caregiver, you are My precious child. I love you just the way you are, a dedicated caregiver who may be tired, lonely, angry, questioning, and guilt-laden. In My arms you will always find refuge and rest. I proved My love for you when I sent My Son to die on the cross and overcome death. That is assurance as we walk this caregiving season together.

I shall not want.

My precious lamb, My grace will always be

sufficient for every step you take. My Holy Word will nourish you. My continual presence will be your strength and hope. Out of My love I will give you resources to help with your loved one—professional caregivers, counselors, family, friends, and more. Look for My blessings interlaced throughout your day!

He makes me lie down in green pastures. He leads me beside still waters. He restores my soul.

Pour out your heart to Me, and then be still and know that I am God. Spending time with Me, your heavenly caregiver, will always renew your attitude and refresh your soul with everlasting hope! Be assured that My mercies will be new each morning, no matter how heavy your burdens.

He leads me in paths of righteousness for His name's sake.

I love being with you, My lamb. You will recognize My voice as we spend time together. Throughout the many challenges, choices, and changes you face as a caregiver, I will be there guiding, leading, and comforting you.

Even though I walk through the valley of the shadow of death, I will fear no evil, for You are with me; Your rod and Your staff, they comfort me.

As your almighty caregiver, I know the valleys you walk through. Not one detail about you, My beloved lamb, goes unnoticed. At times you may doubt that My plans for you are good and full of hope, but I am in control. Trust My faithfulness!

You prepare a table before me in the presence of my enemies; You anoint my head with oil; my cup overflows.

I take great delight in you. I look forward to having you sit at My banqueting table each time you feast on My Word and commune with Me. As your shepherd, I am your refuge. Doubt and discouragement, your enemies, are powerless. The oil of My blessings will overflow, and you will know a peace that passes all understanding.

Surely goodness and mercy shall follow me all the days of my life, and I shall dwell in the house of the LORD forever.

Look to Me as your caregiver. I love you! I have redeemed you! Let Me be your firm foundation as you walk through the valleys of disappointment and green pastures of rest. I will never leave you nor forsake you, for in Me you have the guarantee of eternal life.

I am the Good Shepherd. Follow Me!

Scripture

EXODUS 4:10, 12

But Moses said to the LORD,
"Oh, my Lord, I am not eloquent,
either in the past or since You have spoken
to Your servant, but I am slow of speech
and of tongue." Then the LORD said to
him, . . . "Go, and I will be with your mouth
and teach you what you shall speak."

EXODUS 33:14

And He said, "My presence will
go with you, and I will give you rest."

DEUTERONOMY 31:6

"Be strong and courageous. Do
not fear or be in dread of them, for it is
the LORD your God who goes with you.
He will not leave you or forsake you."

PROVERBS 3:5–6

Trust in the LORD with all your
heart, and do not lean on your own understanding. In all your ways acknowledge
Him, and He will make straight your paths.

Matthew 6:34 NIV

Therefore, do not worry about tomorrow, for tomorrow will worry about itself. Each day has enough trouble of its own.

Matthew 11:28–30

"Come to Me, all who labor and are heavy laden, and I will give you rest. Take My yoke upon you, and learn from Me, for I am gentle and lowly in heart, and you will find rest for your souls. For My yoke is easy, and My burden is light."

Matthew 14:27

But immediately Jesus spoke to them, saying, "Take heart; it is I. Do not be afraid."

John 3:16–17

For God so loved the world, that He gave His only Son, that whoever believes in Him should not perish but have eternal life. For God did not send His Son into the world to condemn the world, but in order that the world might be saved through Him.

1 Corinthians 12:22, 24

The parts of the body that seem
to be weaker are indispensable . . . God
has so composed the body, giving greater honor to the part that lacked it.

2 Corinthians 1:3–4

Blessed be the God and Father
of our Lord Jesus Christ, the Father of
mercies and God of all comfort, who
comforts us in all our affliction, so that we
may be able to comfort those who are in
any affliction, with the comfort with which
we ourselves are comforted by God.

2 Corinthians 4:17–18

For this light momentary
affliction is preparing for us an eternal
weight of glory beyond all comparison,
as we look not to the things that are seen
but to the things that are unseen. For
the things that are seen are transient,
but the things that are unseen are eternal.

Philippians 2:4

Let each of you look not only to his own interests, but also to the interests of others.

Hebrews 13:5b–6, 8

"I will never leave you nor forsake you." So we can confidently say, "The Lord is my helper; I will not fear; what can man do to me?" . . . Jesus Christ is the same yesterday and today and forever.

James 1:12

Blessed is the man who remains steadfast under trial, for when he has stood the test he will receive the crown of life, which God has promised to those who love Him.

1 Peter 1:6–9 NIV

In this you greatly rejoice, though now for a little while you may have had to suffer grief in all kinds of trials. These have come so that your faith—of greater worth than gold, which perishes even though refined by fire—may be proved genuine and may result in praise, glory and honor when Jesus

Christ is revealed. Though you have not seen Him, you love Him; and even though you do not see Him now, you believe in Him and are filled with an inexpressible and glorious joy, for you are receiving the goal of your faith, the salvation of your souls.

1 PETER 3:4

But let your adorning be the hidden person of the heart with the imperishable beauty of a gentle and quiet spirit, which in God's sight is very precious.

1 PETER 3:8, 12–14a

Finally, all of you, have unity of mind, sympathy, brotherly love, a tender heart, and a humble mind. . . . "For the eyes of the Lord are on the righteous, and His ears are open to their prayer." . . . Now who is there to harm you if you are zealous for what is good? But even if you should suffer for righteousness sake, you will be blessed.

1 JOHN 3:16–18

By this we know love, that He laid down His life for us, and we ought to lay down our lives for the brothers. But if anyone has the world's goods and sees his brother in need, yet closes his heart against him, how does God's love abide in him? Little children, let us not love in word or talk but in deed and in truth.

1 JOHN 4:7–12

Beloved, let us love one another, for love is from God, and whoever loves has been born of God and knows God. Anyone who does not love does not know God, because God is love. In this the love of God was made manifest among us, that God sent His only Son into the world, so that we might live through Him. In this is love, not that we have loved God but that He loved us and sent His Son to be the propitiation for our sins. Beloved, if God so loved us, we also ought to love one another. No one has ever seen God; if we love one another, God abides in us and His love is perfected in us.

Psalms

PSALM 4:1, 6–8

Faith

Answer me when I call, O God of my
   righteousness!
You have given me relief when I was in distress.
Be gracious to me and hear my prayer! ...

There are many who say, "Who will show
   us some good?
   Lift up the light of Your face upon us,
   O LORD!"
You have put more joy in my heart than they
   have when their grain and wine abound.

In peace I will both lie down and sleep;
   for You alone, O LORD, make me dwell
   in safety.

PSALM 8

God's Majesty

O LORD, our Lord,
   how majestic is Your name in all the earth!
You have set Your glory above the heavens.

Out of the mouth of babies and infants,
You have established strength because
of Your foes,
to still the enemy and the avenger.

When I look at Your heavens, the work
of Your fingers,
the moon and the stars, which You
have set in place,
what is man that You are mindful of him,
and the son of man that you care for him?

Yet You have made him a little lower than
the heavenly beings
and crowned him with glory and honor.
You have given him dominion over the
works of Your hands;
You have put all things under his feet,
all sheep and oxen,
and also the beasts of the field,
the birds of the heavens, and the fish
of the sea,
whatever passes along the paths of the
seas.

O LORD, our Lord,
how majestic is Your name in all the earth!

Psalm 9:9–10
Strength

The LORD is a stronghold for the oppressed,
   a stronghold in times of trouble.
And those who know Your name put their
         trust in You,
      for You, O LORD, have not forsaken
         those who seek You.

Psalm 16:11
Refuge

You make known to me the path of life;
   in Your presence there is fullness of joy;
   at Your right hand are pleasures
         forevermore.

Psalm 23
Trust

The LORD is my shepherd; I shall not want.
   He makes me lie down in green
         pastures.
He leads me beside still waters.
   He restores my soul.
He leads me in paths of righteousness
   for His name's sake.

Even though I walk through the valley of the
    shadow of death,
    I will fear no evil,
for You are with me;
    Your rod and Your staff,
    they comfort me.

You prepare a table before me
    in the presence of my enemies;
You anoint my head with oil;
    my cup overflows.
Surely goodness and mercy shall follow me
    all the days of my life,
and I shall dwell in the house of the LORD
    forever.

PSALM 31:14–16

Trust

But I trust in You, O LORD;
    I say, "You are my God."
My times are in Your hand;
    rescue me from the hand of my enemies
        and from my persecutors!
Make Your face shine on Your servant;
    save me in Your steadfast love!

PSALM 32

Forgiveness

Blessed is the one whose transgression is
     forgiven,
     whose sin is covered.
Blessed is the man against whom the LORD
     counts no iniquity,
     and in whose spirit there is no deceit.

For when I kept silent, my bones wasted away
     through my groaning all day long.
For day and night Your hand was heavy
     upon me;
     my strength was dried up as by the heat
     of summer.
                                        Selah

I acknowledged my sin to You,
     and I did not cover my iniquity;
I said, "I will confess my transgressions
     to the LORD,"
     and You forgave the iniquity of my sin.
                                        Selah

Therefore let everyone who is godly
     offer prayer to You at a time
     when You may be found;

surely in the rush of great waters,
    they shall not reach him.
You are a hiding place for me;
    You preserve me from trouble;
    You surround me with shouts of
        deliverance.

Selah

I will instruct you and teach you in the way
    you should go;
    I will counsel you with my eye upon you.
Be not like a horse or a mule, without
    understanding,
    which must be curbed with bit and bridle,
    or it will not stay near you.
Many are the sorrows of the wicked,
    but steadfast love surrounds the
        one who trusts in the LORD.
Be glad in the LORD, and rejoice,
    O righteous,
    and shout for joy, all you upright in heart!

PSALM 34:1–5, 8–10, 19–20, 22
Deliverance

I will bless the LORD at all times;
    His praise shall continu-
    ally be in my mouth.

My soul makes its boast in the LORD;
    let the humble hear and be glad.
Oh, magnify the LORD with me,
    and let us exalt His name together!

I sought the LORD, and He answered me
    and delivered me from all my fears.
Those who look to Him are radiant,
    and their faces shall never be
        ashamed. . . .

Oh, taste and see that the LORD is good!
    Blessed is the man who
        takes refuge in Him!
Oh, fear the LORD, you His saints,
    for those who fear Him have no lack!
The young lions suffer want and hunger;
    but those who seek the LORD
        lack no good thing. . . .

Many are the afflictions of the righteous,
    but the LORD delivers him out of them all.
He keeps all his bones;
    not one of them is broken. . . .
The LORD redeems the life of His servants;
    none of those who take refuge
        in Him will be condemned.

Psalm 42:11

Hope

Why are you cast down, O my soul,
    and why are you in turmoil within me?
Hope in God; for I shall again praise Him,
    my salvation and my God.

Psalm 46:1–3, 10–11

Strength

God is our refuge and strength,
    a very present help in trouble.
Therefore we will not fear though the earth
      gives way,
    though the mountains be moved into the
      heart of the sea,
though its waters roar and foam,
    though the mountains tremble at
      its swelling.

Selah . . .

"Be still, and know that I am God.
    I will be exalted among the nations,
    I will be exalted in the earth!"
The LORD of hosts is with us;
    the God of Jacob is our fortress.

Selah

PSALM 55:1–2, 5-8, 16–18a, 22

Anguish and Redemption

Give ear to my prayer, O God,
  and hide not Yourself from my plea for
    mercy!
Attend to me, and answer me;
  I am restless in my complaint
    and I moan, . . .

Fear and trembling come upon me,
  and horror overwhelms me.
And I say, "Oh, that I had wings like a dove!
  I would fly away and be at rest;
yes, I would wander far away;
  I would lodge in the wilderness;

Selah

I would hurry to find a shelter
  from the raging wind and tempest." . . .

But I call to God,
  and the LORD will save me.
Evening and morning and at noon
  I utter my complaint and moan,
  and He hears my voice.
He redeems my soul . . .

Cast your burden on the LORD,
 and He will sustain you;
He will never permit
 the righteous to be moved.

PSALM 62:5–8

Hope and Refuge

For God alone, O my soul, wait in silence,
 for my hope is from Him.
He only is my rock and my salvation,
 my fortress; I shall not be shaken.
On God rests my salvation and my glory;
 my mighty rock, my refuge is God.
Trust in Him at all times, O people;
 pour out your heart before Him;
 God is a refuge for us.

Selah

PSALM 63:1–8

Steadfast Love

O God, You are my God; earnestly I seek You;
 my soul thirsts for You;
my flesh faints for You,
 as in a dry and weary land where there is
  no water.
So I have looked upon You in the sanctuary,

beholding Your power and glory.
Because Your steadfast love is better than life,
　　my lips will praise You.

So I will bless You as long as I live;
　　in Your name I will lift up my hands.
My soul will be satisfied as with fat and
　　　rich food,
　　and my mouth will praise You with
　　　joyful lips,
when I remember You upon my bed,
　　and meditate on You in the watches
　　　of the night;
for You have been my help,
　　and in the shadow of Your wings I will
　　　sing for joy.
My soul clings to You;
　　Your right hand upholds me.

PSALM 84

Praise

How lovely is Your dwelling place,
　　O LORD of hosts!
My soul longs, yes, faints
　　for the courts of the LORD;
my heart and flesh sing for joy
　　to the living God.

Even the sparrow finds a home,
  and the swallow a nest for herself,
  where she may lay her young,
at your altars, O LORD of hosts,
  my King and my God.
Blessed are those who dwell in Your house,
  ever singing Your praise!

Selah

Blessed are those whose strength is in You,
  in whose heart are the highways to Zion.
As they go through the Valley of Baca
  they make it a place of springs;
  the early rain also covers it with pools.
They go from strength to strength;
  each one appears before God in Zion.
O LORD God of hosts, hear my prayer;
  give ear, O God of Jacob!

Selah

Behold our shield, O God;
  look on the face of Your anointed!
For a day in Your courts is better
  than a thousand elsewhere.
I would rather be a doorkeeper in the house
    of my God
  than dwell in the tents of wickedness.

For the Lord God is a sun and shield;
    the Lord bestows favor and honor.
No good thing does He withhold
    from those who walk uprightly.
O Lord of hosts,
    blessed is the one who trusts in You!

Psalm 86:1–7

Grace

Incline Your ear, O Lord, and answer me,
    for I am poor and needy.
Preserve my life, for I am godly;
    save Your servant, who trusts
        in You—You are my God.
Be gracious to me, O Lord,
    for to You do I cry all the day.
Gladden the soul of Your servant,
    for to You, O Lord, do I lift up my soul.
For You, O Lord, are good and forgiving,
    abounding in steadfast love to
        all who call upon You.
Give ear, O Lord, to my prayer;
    listen to my plea for grace.
In the day of my trouble I call upon You,
    for You answer me.

PSALM 91:1–2, 11–12, 14–16
Refuge and Fortress

He who dwells in the shelter of the
  Most High
  will abide in the shadow of the Almighty.
I will say to the LORD, "My refuge and my
  fortress,
  my God, in whom I trust." . . .

For He will command His angels
  concerning you
  to guard you in all your ways.
On their hands they will bear you up,
  lest you strike your foot against a stone. . . .

"Because he holds fast to Me in love, I will
  deliver him;
  I will protect him, because he knows
  My name.
When he calls to Me, I will answer him;
  I will be with him in trouble;
  I will rescue him and honor him.
With long life I will satisfy him
  and show him My salvation."

Psalm 100

Joy

Make a joyful noise to the LORD,
>   all the earth!
>   Serve the LORD with gladness!
>   Come into His presence with singing!

Know that the LORD, He is God!
>   It is He who made us, and we are His;
>   we are His people, and the
>   sheep of His pasture.

Enter His gates with thanksgiving,
>   and His courts with praise!
>   Give thanks to Him; bless His name!

For the LORD is good;
>   His steadfast love endures forever,
>   and His faithfulness to all generations.

Psalm 116:1–2, 5–9, 12–13

Mercy

I love the LORD, because He has heard
>   my voice and my pleas for mercy.
Because He inclined His ear to me,
>   therefore I will call on Him
>   as long as I live. . . .

Gracious is the LORD, and righteous;
    our God is merciful.
The LORD preserves the simple;
    when I was brought low, He saved me.
Return, O my soul, to your rest;
    for the LORD has dealt boun-
      tifully with you.

For You have delivered my soul from death,
    my eyes from tears,
    my feet from stumbling;
I will walk before the LORD
    in the land of the living. . . .

What shall I render to the LORD
    for all His benefits to me?
I will lift up the cup of salvation
    and call on the name of the LORD.

PSALM 117

Faithfulness

Praise the LORD, all nations!
    Extol Him, all peoples!
For great is His steadfast love toward us,
    and the faithfulness of the LORD endures
      forever.
Praise the LORD!

Psalm 118:1, 5–6, 22–24, 28–29

Thanksgiving

Oh give thanks to the LORD, for He is good;
  for His steadfast love endures forever! . . .

Out of my distress I called on the LORD;
  the LORD answered me and set me free.
The LORD is on my side; I will not fear.
  What can man do to me? . . .

The stone that the builders rejected
  has become the cornerstone.
This is the LORD's doing;
  it is marvelous in our eyes.
This is the day that the LORD has made;
  let us rejoice and be glad in it. . . .

You are my God, and I will give thanks to
      You;
  You are my God; I will extol You.
Oh give thanks to the LORD, for He is good;
  for His steadfast love endures forever!

Psalm 121

Assurance

I lift up my eyes to the hills.
From where does my help come?
My help comes from the LORD,
who made heaven and earth.

He will not let your foot be moved;
He who keeps you will not slumber.
Behold, He who keeps Israel
will neither slumber nor sleep.

The LORD is your keeper;
the LORD is your shade on your right
hand.
The sun shall not strike you by day,
nor the moon by night.

The LORD will keep you from all evil;
He will keep your life.
The LORD will keep
your going out and your coming in
from this time forth and forevermore.

PSALM 130

Trust in God's Mercy

Out of the depths I cry to You, O LORD!
    O Lord, hear my voice!
Let Your ears be attentive
    to the voice of my pleas for mercy!

If You, O LORD, should mark iniquities,
    O Lord, who could stand?
But with You there is forgiveness,
    that You may be feared.
I wait for the LORD, my soul waits,
    and in His word I hope;
my soul waits for the Lord
    more than watchmen for the morning,
    more than watchmen for the morning.

O Israel, hope in the LORD!
    For with the LORD there is steadfast love,
and with Him is plentiful redemption.
And He will redeem Israel
    from all his iniquities.

PSALM 139:1–6, 23–24

Omnipotent God

O LORD, You have searched
    me and known me!
You know when I sit down and when
    I rise up;
    You discern my thoughts from afar.
You search out my path and my lying down
    and are acquainted with all my ways.
Even before a word is on my tongue,
    behold, O LORD, You know it altogether.
You hem me in, behind and before,
    and lay Your hand upon me.
Such knowledge is too wonderful for me;
    it is high; I cannot attain it. . . .

Search me, O God, and know my heart!
    Try me and know my thoughts!
And see if there be any grievous way in me,
    and lead me in the way everlasting!

A MIGHTY FORTRESS IS OUR GOD

A mighty fortress is our God,
    A trusty shield and weapon;
He helps us free from ev'ry need
    That hath us now o'ertaken.
The old evil foe
Now means deadly woe;
    Deep guile and great might
    Are his dread arms in fight;
On earth is not his equal.

With might of ours can naught be done,
    Soon were our loss effected;
But for us fights the valiant One,
    Whom God Himself elected.
Ask ye, Who is this?
Jesus Christ it is,
    Of Sabaoth Lord,
    And there's none other God;
He holds the field forever.

Though devils all the world should fill,
    All eager to devour us,
We tremble not, we fear no ill;
    They shall not overpow'r us.

This world's prince may still
Scowl fierce as he will,
   He can harm us none.
   He's judged; the deed is done;
One little word can fell him.

The Word they still shall let remain
   Nor any thanks have for it;
He's by our side upon the plain
   With His good gifts and Spirit.
And take they our life,
Goods, fame, child, and wife,
   Though these all be gone,
   Our vict'ry has been won;
The Kingdom ours remaineth.
(*LSB* 656)

Abide with Me

Abide with me, fast falls the eventide.
The darkness deepens; Lord, with me abide.
When other helpers fail and comforts flee,
Help of the helpless, O abide with me.

I need Thy presence ev'ry passing hour;
What but Thy grace can foil
   the tempter's pow'r?
Who like Thyself my guide and stay can be?

Through cloud and sunshine,
    O abide with me.
Come not in terrors, as the King of kings,
But kind and good, with healing in Thy wings;
Tears for all woes, a heart for ev'ry plea.
Come, Friend of sinners, thus abide with me.

Swift to its close ebbs out life's little day;
Earth's joys grow dim, its glories pass away;
Change and decay in all around I see;
O Thou who changest not, abide with me.

I fear no foe with Thee at hand to bless;
Ills have no weight and tears no bitterness.
Where is death's sting? Where,
    grave, thy victory?
I triumph still if Thou abide with me!

Hold Thou Thy cross before my closing eyes;
Shine through the gloom, and
    point me to the skies.
Heav'n's morning breaks, and
    earth's vain shadows flee;
In life, in death, O Lord, abide with me.

(*LSB* 878)

AMAZING GRACE

Amazing grace—how sweet the sound—
    That saved a wretch like me!
I once was lost but now am found,
    Was blind but now I see!

The Lord has promised good to me,
    His Word my hope secures;
He will my shield and portion be
    As long as life endures.

Through many dangers, toils, and snares
    I have already come;
His grace has brought me safe thus far,
    His grace will lead me home.

Yes, when this flesh and heart shall fail
    And mortal life shall cease,
Amazing grace shall then prevail
    In heaven's joy and peace.

When we've been there ten thousand years,
    Bright shining as the sun,
We've no less days to sing God's praise
    Than when we'd first begun.

(*LSB* 744)

BEAUTIFUL SAVIOR

Beautiful Savior,
King of creation,
Son of God and Son of Man!
Truly I'd love Thee,
Truly I'd serve Thee,
Light of my soul, my joy, my crown.

Fair are the meadows,
Fair are the woodlands,
Robed in flow'rs of blooming spring;
Jesus is fairer,
Jesus is purer,
He makes our sorr'wing spirit sing.

Fair is the sunshine,
Fair is the moonlight,
Bright the sparkling stars on high;
Jesus shines brighter,
Jesus shines purer
Than all the angels in the sky.

Beautiful Savior,
Lord of the nations,
Son of God and Son of Man!

Glory and honor,
　　Praise, adoration
Now and forevermore be Thine!
(*LSB* 537)

COME UNTO ME, YE WEARY

"Come unto Me, ye weary,
　　And I will give you rest."
O blessèd voice of Jesus,
　　Which comes to hearts oppressed!
It tells of benediction,
　　Of pardon, grace, and peace,
Of joy that hath no ending,
　　Of love that cannot cease.

"Come unto Me, ye wand'rers,
　　And I will give you light."
O loving voice of Jesus,
　　Which comes to cheer the night!
Our hearts were filled with sadness,
　　And we had lost our way;
But Thou hast brought us gladness
　　And songs at break of day.

"Come unto Me, ye fainting,
　　And I will give you life."
O cheering voice of Jesus,

Which comes to aid our strife!
The foe is stern and eager,
    The fight is fierce and long;
But Thou hast made us mighty
    And stronger than the strong.

"And whosoever cometh,
    I will not cast him out."
O patient love of Jesus,
    Which drives away our doubt,
Which, though we be unworthy
    Of love so great and free,
Invites us very sinners
    To come, dear Lord, to Thee!
(LSB 684)

Go, My Children, with My Blessing

Go, My children, with My blessing,
    Never alone.
Waking, sleeping, I am with you;
    You are My own.
    In My love's baptismal river
    I have made you Mine forever.
Go, My children, with My blessing—
    You are My own.

Go, My children, fed and nourished,
    Closer to Me;
Grow in love and love by serving,
    Joyful and free.
  Here My Spirit's power filled you;
  Here His tender comfort stilled you.
Go, My children, fed and nourished,
    Joyful and free.

I the Lord will bless and keep you
    And give you peace;
I the Lord will smile upon you
    And give you peace:
  I the Lord will be your Father,
  Savior, Comforter, and Brother.
Go, My children; I will keep you
    And give you peace.

(*LSB* 922:1, 3, 4)

GOD LOVED THE WORLD SO THAT HE GAVE

God loved the world so that He gave
His only Son the lost to save,
That all who would in Him believe
Should everlasting life receive.

Christ Jesus is the ground of faith,
Who was made flesh and suffered death;
All then who trust in Him alone
Are built on this chief cornerstone.

God would not have the sinner die;
His Son with saving grace is nigh;
His Spirit in the Word declares
How we in Christ are heaven's heirs.

Be of good cheer, for God's own Son
Forgives all sins which you have done;
And, justified by Jesus' blood,
Your Baptism grants the highest good.

If you are sick, if death is near,
This truth your troubled heart can cheer:
Christ Jesus saves your soul from death;
That is the firmest ground of faith.

Glory to God the Father, Son,
And Holy Spirit, Three in One!
To You, O blessèd Trinity,
Be praise now and eternally!

(*LSB* 571)

GOD LOVES ME DEARLY

God loves me dearly,
Grants me salvation,
God loves me dearly,
Loves even me. *Refrain*

Refrain:
Therefore I'll say again:
God loves me dearly,
God loves me dearly,
Loves even me.

I was in slav'ry,
Sin, death, and darkness;
God's love was working
To make me free. *Refrain*

He sent forth Jesus,
My dear Redeemer,
He sent forth Jesus
And set me free. *Refrain*

Jesus, my Savior,
Himself did offer;
Jesus, my Savior,
Paid all I owed. *Refrain*

Now I will praise You,
O Love Eternal;
Now I will praise You
All my life long. *Refrain*
(*LSB* 392)

HAVE NO FEAR, LITTLE FLOCK

Have no fear, little flock;
Have no fear, little flock,
    For the Father has chosen
    To give you the Kingdom;
Have no fear, little flock!

Have good cheer, little flock;
Have good cheer, little flock,
    For the Father will keep you
    In His love forever;
Have good cheer, little flock!

Praise the Lord high above;
Praise the Lord high above,
    For He stoops down to heal you,
    Uplift and restore you;
Praise the Lord high above!

Thankful hearts raise to God;
Thankful hearts raise to God,

For He stays close beside you,
In all things works with you;
Thankful hearts raise to God!
(*LSB* 735)

How Sweet the Name of Jesus Sounds

How sweet the name of Jesus sounds
In a believer's ear!
It soothes our sorrows, heals our wounds,
And drives away our fear.

It makes the wounded spirit whole
And calms the heart's unrest;
'Tis manna to the hungry soul
And to the weary, rest.

Dear name! The rock on which I build,
My shield and hiding place;
My never-failing treasury filled
With boundless stores of grace.

O Jesus, shepherd, guardian, friend,
My Prophet, Priest, and King,
My Lord, my life, my way, my end,
Accept the praise I bring.

How weak the effort of my heart,
    How cold my warmest thought!
But when I see Thee as Thou art,
    I'll praise Thee as I ought.

Till then I would Thy love proclaim
    With ev'ry fleeting breath;
And may the music of Thy name
    Refresh my soul in death!
(*LSB* 524)

I AM JESUS' LITTLE LAMB

I am Jesus' little lamb,
Ever glad at heart I am;
For my Shepherd gently guides me,
Knows my need and well provides me,
Loves me ev'ry day the same,
Even calls me by my name.

Day by day, at home, away,
Jesus is my staff and stay.
When I hunger, Jesus feeds me,
Into pleasant pastures leads me;
When I thirst, He bids me go
Where the quiet waters flow.

Who so happy as I am,
Even now the Shepherd's lamb?
And when my short life is ended,
By His angel host attended,
He shall fold me to His breast,
There within His arms to rest.

(*LSB* 740)

I Am Trusting Thee, Lord Jesus

I am trusting Thee, Lord Jesus,
    Trusting only Thee;
Trusting Thee for full salvation,
    Great and free.

I am trusting Thee for pardon;
    At Thy feet I bow,
For Thy grace and tender mercy
    Trusting now.

I am trusting Thee for cleansing
    In the crimson flood;
Trusting Thee to make me holy
    By Thy blood.

I am trusting Thee to guide me;
    Thou alone shalt lead,

Ev'ry day and hour supplying
    All my need.

I am trusting Thee for power;
    Thine can never fail.
Words which Thou Thyself shalt give me
    Must prevail.

I am trusting Thee, Lord Jesus;
    Never let me fall.
I am trusting Thee forever
    And for all.

(*LSB* 729)

I HEARD THE VOICE OF JESUS SAY

I heard the voice of Jesus say,
    "Come unto Me and rest;
Lay down, thou weary one, lay down
    Thy head upon My breast."
I came to Jesus as I was,
    So weary, worn, and sad;
I found in Him a resting place,
    And He has made me glad.

I heard the voice of Jesus say,
    "Behold, I freely give

The living water; thirsty one,
    Stoop down and drink and live."
I came to Jesus, and I drank
    Of that life-giving stream;
My thirst was quenched, my soul revived,
    And now I live in Him.

I heard the voice of Jesus say,
    "I am this dark world's light.
Look unto Me; thy morn shall rise
    And all thy day be bright."
I looked to Jesus, and I found
    In Him my star, my sun;
And in that light of life I'll walk
    Till trav'ling days are done.

(*LSB* 699)

I'M BUT A STRANGER HERE

I'm but a stranger here,
    Heav'n is my home;
Earth is a desert drear,
    Heav'n is my home.
Danger and sorrow stand
Round me on ev'ry hand;
Heav'n is my fatherland,
    Heav'n is my home.

What though the tempest rage,
  Heav'n is my home;
Short is my pilgrimage,
  Heav'n is my home;
And time's wild wintry blast
Soon shall be overpast;
I shall reach home at last,
  Heav'n is my home.

Therefore I murmur not,
  Heav'n is my home;
Whate'er my earthly lot,
  Heav'n is my home;
And I shall surely stand
There at my Lord's right hand;
Heav'n is my fatherland,
  Heav'n is my home.

(*LSB* 748)

In Thee Is Gladness

In Thee is gladness
Amid all sadness,
Jesus, sunshine of my heart.
By Thee are given
The gifts of heaven,
Thou the true Redeemer art.
Our souls Thou wakest,

Our bonds Thou breakest;
  Who trusts Thee surely
  Has built securely;
He stands forever: Alleluia!
  Our hearts are pining
  To see Thy shining,
  Dying or living
  To Thee are cleaving;
Naught can us sever: Alleluia!

  Since He is ours,
  We fear no powers,
Not of earth nor sin nor death.
  He sees and blesses
  In worst distresses;
He can change them with a breath.
  Wherefore the story
  Tell of His glory
  With hearts and voices;
  All heav'n rejoices
In Him forever: Alleluia!
  We shout for gladness,
  Triumph o'er sadness,
  Love Him and praise Him
  And still shall raise Him
Glad hymns forever: Alleluia!

(*LSB* 818)

JESUS LOVES ME

Jesus loves me! This I know,
For the Bible tells me so.
Little ones to Him belong;
They are weak, but He is strong.

Refrain:
Yes, Jesus loves me!
Yes, Jesus loves me!
Yes, Jesus loves me!
The Bible tells me so.

Jesus loves me! He who died
Heaven's gates to open wide.
He has washed away my sin,
Lets His little child come in. *Refrain*
(*LSB* 588)

JESUS, SAVIOR, PILOT ME

Jesus, Savior, pilot me
Over life's tempestuous sea;
Unknown waves before me roll,
Hiding rock and treach'rous shoal.
Chart and compass come from Thee.
Jesus, Savior, pilot me.

As a mother stills her child,
Thou canst hush the ocean wild;
   Boist'rous waves obey Thy will
   When Thou say'st to them, "Be still!"
Wondrous Sov'reign of the sea,
Jesus, Savior, pilot me.

When at last I near the shore
And the fearful breakers roar
   Twixt me and the peaceful rest,
   Then, while leaning on the Thy breast,
May I hear Thee say to me,
"Fear not, I will pilot thee."
(*LSB* 715)

JESUS, THY BLOOD AND RIGHTEOUSNESS

Jesus, Thy blood and righteousness
My beauty are, my glorious dress;
Midst flaming worlds, in these arrayed,
With joy shall I lift up my head.
Bold shall I stand in that great day,
Cleansed and redeemed, no debt to pay;
Fully absolved through these I am
From sin and fear, from guilt and shame.

Lord, I believe Thy precious blood,
Which at the mercy seat of God
Pleads for the captives' liberty,
Was also shed in love for me.

Lord, I believe, were sinners more
Than sands upon the ocean shore,
Thou hast for all a ransom paid,
For all a full atonement made.
When from the dust of death I rise
To claim my mansion in the skies,
This then shall be my only plea:
Jesus hath lived and died for me.

Jesus, be endless praise to Thee,
Whose boundless mercy hath for me,
For me, and all Thy hands have made,
An everlasting ransom paid.
(*LSB* 563)

JUST AS I AM, WITHOUT ONE PLEA

Just as I am, without one plea
But that Thy blood was shed for me
And that Thou bidd'st me come to Thee,
   O Lamb of God, I come, I come.

Just as I am and waiting not
To rid my soul of one dark blot,
To Thee, whose blood can cleanse each spot,
   O Lamb of God, I come, I come.

Just as I am, though tossed about
With many a conflict, many a doubt,
Fightings and fears within, without,
   O Lamb of God, I come, I come.

Just as I am, poor, wretched, blind;
Sight, riches, healing of the mind,
Yea, all I need, in Thee to find,
   O Lamb of God, I come, I come.

Just as I am, Thou wilt receive,
Wilt welcome, pardon, cleanse, relieve;
Because Thy promise I believe,
   O Lamb of God, I come, I come.

Just as I am; Thy love unknown
Has broken ev'ry barrier down;
Now to be Thine, yea, Thine alone,
   O Lamb of God, I come, I come.

(LSB 570)

LET US EVER WALK WITH JESUS

Let us ever walk with Jesus,
　　Follow His example pure,
Through a world that would deceive us
　　And to sin our spirits lure.
Onward in His footsteps treading,
　　Pilgrims here, our home above,
　　Full of faith and hope and love,
Let us do the Father's bidding.
　　Faithful Lord, with me abide;
　　I shall follow where You guide.

Let us suffer here with Jesus
　　And with patience bear our cross.
Joy will follow all our sadness;
　　Where He is, there is no loss.
Though today we sow no laughter,
　　We shall reap celestial joy;
　　All discomforts that annoy
Shall give way to mirth hereafter.
　　Jesus, here I share Your woe;
　　Help me there Your joy to know.
Let us also live with Jesus.
　　He has risen from the dead
That to life we may awaken.
　　Jesus, You are now our head.

We are Your own living members;
    Where You live, there we shall be
    In Your presence constantly,
Living there with You forever.
    Jesus, let me faithful be,
    Life eternal grant to me.

(LSB 685:1, 2, 4) Copyright © 1978
Lutheran Book of Worship

LORD, TAKE MY HAND AND LEAD ME

Lord, take my hand and lead me
    Upon life's way;
Direct, protect, and feed me
    From day to day.
Without Your grace and favor
    I go astray;
So take my hand, O Savior,
    And lead the way.

Lord, when the tempest rages,
    I need not fear,
For You, the Rock of Ages,
    Are always near.
Close by Your side abiding,
    I fear no foe,
For when Your hand is guiding,
    In peace I go.

Lord, when the shadows lengthen
   And night has come,
I know that You will strengthen
   My steps toward home.
Then nothing can impede me,
   O blessèd Friend;
So take my hand and lead me
   Unto the end.

My Faith Looks Up to Thee

My faith looks up to Thee,
Thou Lamb of Calvary,
   Savior divine.
Now hear me while I pray;
Take all my guilt away;
O let me from this day
   Be wholly Thine!

May Thy rich grace impart
Strength to my fainting heart;
   My zeal inspire!
As Thou hast died for me,
Oh, may my love to Thee
Pure, warm, and changeless be,
   A living fire!

While life's dark maze I tread
And griefs around me spread,
   Be Thou my guide;
Bid darkness turn to day,
Wipe sorrow's tears away,
Nor let me ever stray
   From Thee aside.

When ends life's transient dream,
When death's cold, sullen stream
   Shall o'er me roll,
Blest Savior, then, in love,
Fear and distrust remove;
O bear me safe above,
   A ransomed soul!

(*LSB* 702)

MY HOPE IS BUILT ON NOTHING LESS

My hope is built on nothing less
Than Jesus' blood and righteousness;
No merit of my own I claim
But wholly lean on Jesus' name.

Refrain:
On Christ, the solid rock, I stand;
All other ground is sinking sand.

When darkness veils His lovely face,
I rest on His unchanging grace;
In ev'ry high and stormy gale
My anchor holds within the veil. *Refrain*

His oath, His covenant and blood
Support me in the raging flood;
When ev'ry earthly prop gives way,
He then is all my hope and stay. *Refrain*

When He shall come with trumpet sound,
Oh, may I then in Him be found,
Clothed in His righteousness alone,
Redeemed to stand before
   His throne! *Refrain*

(*LSB* 575)

NOW THE LIGHT HAS GONE AWAY

Now the light has gone away;
Father, listen while I pray,
Asking Thee to watch and keep
And to send me quiet sleep.

Jesus, Savior, wash away
All that has been wrong today;
Help me ev'ry day to be
Good and gentle, more like Thee.

Let my near and dear ones be
Always near and dear to Thee;
O bring me and all I love
To Thy happy home above.

Now my evening praise I give;
Thou didst die that I might live.
All my blessings come from Thee;
Oh, how good Thou art to me!

Thou, my best and kindest Friend,
Thou wilt love me to the end.
Let me love Thee more and more,
Always better than before.

(*LSB* 887)

O God, Forsake Me Not

O God, forsake me not!
    Your gracious presence lend me;
Lord, lead Your helpless child;
    Your Holy Spirit send me
That I my course may run.
    O be my light, my lot,
My staff, my rock, my shield—
    O God, forsake me not!

(*LSB* 731:1)

Praise to You and Adoration

> Praise to You and adoration,
>> Blessèd Jesus, Son of God,
> Who, to serve Your own creation,
>> Came to share our flesh and blood.
> Guide me that I never may
> From Your fold or pastures stray,
>> But with zeal and joy exceeding
>> Follow where Your steps are leading.
> Hold me ever in Your keeping;
>> Comfort me in pain and strife.
> In my laughter and my weeping
>> Be with me throughout my life.
> Give me greater love for You,
> And my faith and hope renew
>> In Your birth, Your life, and passion,
>> In Your death and resurrection.

(*LSB* 692)

Rock of Ages, Cleft for Me

> Rock of Ages, cleft for me,
> Let me hide myself in Thee;
> Let the water and the blood,
> From Thy riven side which flowed,
> Be of sin the double cure:
> Cleanse me from its guilt and pow'r.

Not the labors of my hands
Can fulfill Thy Law's demands;
Could my zeal no respite know,
Could my tears forever flow,
All for sin could not atone;
Thou must save, and Thou alone.

Nothing in my hand I bring;
Simply to Thy cross I cling.
Naked, come to Thee for dress;
Helpless, look to Thee for grace;
Foul, I to the fountain fly;
Wash me, Savior, or I die.

While I draw this fleeting breath,
When mine eyelids close in death,
When I soar to worlds unknown,
See Thee on Thy judgment throne,
Rock of Ages, cleft for me,
Let me hide myself in Thee.

(LSB 761)

TAKE MY LIFE AND LET IT BE

Take my life and let it be
Consecrated, Lord, to Thee;
Take my moments and my days,

Let them flow in ceaseless praise.
Take my hands and let them move
At the impulse of Thy love;
Take my feet and let them be
Swift and beautiful for Thee.

Take my voice and let me sing
Always, only for my King;
Take my lips and let them be
Filled with messages from Thee.

Take my silver and my gold,
Not a mite would I withhold;
Take my intellect and use
Ev'ry pow'r as Thou shalt choose.

Take my will and make it Thine,
It shall be no longer mine;
Take my heart, it is Thine own,
It shall be Thy royal throne.

Take my love, my Lord, I pour
At Thy feet its treasure store;
Take myself, and I will be
Ever, only, all for Thee.

(*LSB* 783)

WHAT A FRIEND WE HAVE IN JESUS

What a friend we have in Jesus,
    All our sins and griefs to bear!
What a privilege to carry
    Ev'rything to God in prayer!
Oh, what peace we often forfeit;
    Oh, what needless pain we bear—
All because we do not carry
    Ev'rything to God in prayer!

Have we trials and temptations?
    Is there trouble anywhere?
We should never be discouraged—
    Take it to the Lord in prayer.
Can we find a friend so faithful
    Who will all our sorrows share?
Jesus knows our ev'ry weakness—
    Take it to the Lord in prayer.

Are we weak and heavy laden,
    Cumbered with a load of care?
Precious Savior, still our refuge—
    Take it to the Lord in prayer.
Do thy friends despise, forsake thee?
    Take it to the Lord in prayer.
In His arms He'll take and shield thee;
    Thou wilt find a solace there.

(LSB 770)

WHAT WONDROUS LOVE IS THIS

What wondrous love is this,
   O my soul, O my soul!
What wondrous love is this, O my soul!
   What wondrous love is this
   That caused the Lord of bliss
To bear the dreadful curse for
   my soul, for my soul,
To bear the dreadful curse for my soul!

When I was sinking down, sink-
   ing down, sinking down,
When I was sinking down, sinking down,
   When I was sinking down
   Beneath God's righteous frown,
Christ laid aside His crown for
   my soul, for my soul,
Christ laid aside His crown for my soul.

To God and to the Lamb I
   will sing, I will sing;
To God and to the Lamb I will sing;
   To God and to the Lamb,
   Who is the great I AM,
While millions join the theme,
   I will sing, I will sing,
While millions join the theme, I will sing.

And when from death I'm free,
　I'll sing on, I'll sing on;
And when from death I'm free, I'll sing on.
　And when from death I'm free,
　I'll sing His love for me,
And through eternity I'll sing on, I'll sing on,
And through eternity I'll sing on.

(*LSB* 543)

A BRIEF SUMMARY OF THE
Christian Faith

This is the text of Dr. Martin Luther's Small Catechism, the most popular explanation of the central teachings of the Christian faith. It has been used by countless Christians of all denominations for almost 500 years.

SECTION 1
The Ten Commandments

As the head of the family should teach them in a simple way to his household

THE FIRST COMMANDMENT
You shall have no other gods.

What does this mean? We should fear, love, and trust in God above all things.

THE SECOND COMMANDMENT
You shall not misuse the name of the Lord your God.

What does this mean? We should fear and love God so that we do not curse, swear, use satanic arts, lie, or deceive by His name, but call upon it in every trouble, pray, praise, and give thanks.

THE THIRD COMMANDMENT

Remember the Sabbath day by keeping it holy.

What does this mean? We should fear and love God so that we do not despise preaching and His Word, but hold it sacred and gladly hear and learn it.

THE FOURTH COMMANDMENT

Honor your father and your mother.

What does this mean? We should fear and love God so that we do not despise or anger our parents and other authorities, but honor them, serve and obey them, love and cherish them.

THE FIFTH COMMANDMENT

You shall not murder.

What does this mean? We should fear and love God so that we do not hurt or harm our neighbor in his body, but help and support him in every physical need.

THE SIXTH COMMANDMENT

You shall not commit adultery.

What does this mean? We should fear and love God so that we lead a sexually pure and decent life in what we say and do, and husband and wife love and honor each other.

THE SEVENTH COMMANDMENT

You shall not steal.

What does this mean? We should fear and love God so that we do not take our neighbor's money or possessions, or get them in any dishonest way, but help him to improve and protect his possessions and income.

THE EIGHTH COMMANDMENT

You shall not give false testimony against your neighbor.

What does this mean? We should fear and love God so that we do not tell lies about our neighbor, betray him, slander him, or hurt his reputation, but defend him, speak well of him, and explain everything in the kindest way.

THE NINTH COMMANDMENT

You shall not covet your neighbor's house.

What does this mean? We should fear and love God so that we do not scheme to get our neighbor's inheritance or house, or get it in a way which only appears right, but help and be of service to him in keeping it.

THE TENTH COMMANDMENT

You shall not covet your neighbor's wife, or his manservant or maidservant, his ox or donkey, or anything that belongs to your neighbor.

What does this mean? We should fear and love God so that we do not entice or force away our neighbor's wife, workers, or animals, or turn them against him, but urge them to stay and do their duty.

[The text of the commandments is from **Ex. 20:3, 7, 8, 12–17.**]

THE CLOSE OF THE COMMANDMENTS

What does God say about all these commandments?

He says: "I, the Lord your God, am a jealous God, punishing the children for the sin of the fathers to the third and fourth generation of those who hate Me, but showing love to a thousand generations of those who love Me and keep My commandments." **(Ex. 20:5–6)**

What does this mean? God threatens to punish all who break these commandments. Therefore, we should fear His wrath and not do anything against them. But He promises grace and every blessing to all who keep these commandments. Therefore, we should also love and trust in Him and gladly do what He commands.

The Creed

As the head of the family should teach it in a simple way to his household

THE FIRST ARTICLE

Creation

I believe in God, the Father Almighty, Maker of heaven and earth.

What does this mean? I believe that God has made me and all creatures; that He has given me my body and soul, eyes, ears, and all my members, my reason and all my senses, and still takes care of them.

He also gives me clothing and shoes, food and drink, house and home, wife and children, land, animals, and all I have. He richly and daily provides me with all that I need to support this body and life.

He defends me against all danger and guards and protects me from all evil.

All this He does only out of fatherly, divine goodness and mercy, without any merit or worthiness in me. For all this it is my duty to thank and praise, serve and obey Him.

This is most certainly true.

The Second Article

Redemption

And in Jesus Christ, His only Son, our Lord, who was conceived by the Holy Spirit, born of the Virgin Mary, suffered under Pontius Pilate, was crucified, died and was buried. He descended into hell. The third day He rose again from the dead. He ascended into heaven and sits at the right hand of God, the Father Almighty. From thence He will come to judge the living and the dead.

What does this mean? I believe that Jesus Christ, true God, begotten of the Father from eternity, and also true man, born of the Virgin Mary, is my Lord, who has redeemed me, a lost and condemned person, purchased and won me from all sins, from death, and from the power of the devil; not with gold or silver, but with His holy, precious blood and with His innocent suffering and death, that I may be His own and live under Him in His kingdom and serve Him in everlasting righteousness, innocence, and blessedness, just as He is risen from the dead, lives and reigns to all eternity.

This is most certainly true.

THE THIRD ARTICLE

Sanctification

I believe in the Holy Spirit, the holy Christian church, the communion of saints, the forgiveness of sins, the resurrection of the body, and the life everlasting. Amen.

What does this mean? I believe that I cannot by my own reason or strength believe in Jesus Christ, my Lord, or come to Him; but the Holy Spirit has called me by the Gospel, enlightened me with His gifts, sanctified and kept me in the true faith.

In the same way He calls, gathers, enlightens, and sanctifies the whole Christian church on earth, and keeps it with Jesus Christ in the one true faith.

In this Christian church He daily and richly forgives all my sins and the sins of all believers.

On the Last Day He will raise me and all the dead, and give eternal life to me and all believers in Christ.

This is most certainly true.

The Lord's Prayer

As the head of the family should teach it in a simple way to his household

Our Father who art in heaven, hallowed be Thy name, Thy kingdom come, Thy will be done on earth as it is in heaven. Give us this day our daily bread; and forgive us our trespasses as we forgive those who trespass against us; and lead us not into temptation, but deliver us from evil. For Thine is the kingdom and the power and the glory forever and ever. Amen.

THE INTRODUCTION

Our Father who art in heaven.

What does this mean? With these words God tenderly invites us to believe that He is our true Father and that we are His true children, so that with all boldness and confidence we may ask Him as dear children ask their dear father.

THE FIRST PETITION

Hallowed be Thy name.

What does this mean? God's name is certainly holy in itself, but we pray in this petition that it may be kept holy among us also.

How is God's name kept holy? God's name is kept holy when the Word of God is taught in its truth and purity, and we, as the children of God, also lead holy lives according to it. Help us to do this, dear Father in heaven! But anyone who teaches or lives contrary to God's Word profanes the name of God among us. Protect us from this, heavenly Father!

THE SECOND PETITION

Thy kingdom come.

What does this mean? The kingdom of God certainly comes by itself without our prayer, but we pray in this petition that it may come to us also.

How does God's kingdom come? God's kingdom comes when our heavenly Father gives us His Holy Spirit, so that by His grace we believe His holy Word and lead godly lives here in time and there in eternity.

THE THIRD PETITION

Thy will be done on earth as it is in heaven.

What does this mean? The good and gracious will of God is done even without our prayer, but we pray in this petition that it may be done among us also.

How is God's will done? God's will is done when He breaks and hinders every evil plan and purpose of the devil, the world, and our sinful nature, which do not want us to hallow God's name or let His kingdom come; and when He strengthens and keeps us firm in His Word and faith until we die.

This is His good and gracious will.

THE FOURTH PETITION

Give us this day our daily bread.

What does this mean? God certainly gives daily bread to everyone without our prayers, even to all evil people, but we pray in this petition that God would lead us to realize this and to receive our daily bread with thanksgiving.

What is meant by daily bread? Daily bread includes everything that has to do with the support and needs of the body, such as food, drink, clothing, shoes, house, home, land, animals, money, goods, a devout husband or wife, devout children, devout workers, devout and faithful rulers, good government, good weather, peace, health, self-control, good reputation, good friends, faithful neighbors, and the like.

THE FIFTH PETITION

And forgive us our trespasses as we forgive those who trespass against us.

What does this mean? We pray in this petition that our Father in heaven would not look at our sins, or deny our prayer because of them. We are neither worthy of the things for which we pray, nor have we deserved them, but we ask that He would give them all to us by grace, for we daily sin much and surely deserve nothing but punishment. So we too will sincerely forgive and gladly do good to those who sin against us.

THE SIXTH PETITION

And lead us not into temptation.

What does this mean? God tempts no one. We pray in this petition that God would guard and keep us so that the devil, the world, and our sinful nature may not deceive us or mislead us into false belief, despair, and other great shame and vice. Although we are attacked by these things, we pray that we may finally overcome them and win the victory.

THE SEVENTH PETITION

But deliver us from evil.

What does this mean? We pray in this petition, in summary, that our Father in heaven would rescue us from every evil of body and soul, possessions and reputation, and finally, when our last hour comes, give us a blessed end, and graciously take us from this valley of sorrow to Himself in heaven.

THE CONCLUSION

For Thine is the kingdom and the power and the glory forever and ever. * *Amen.*

What does this mean? This means that I should be certain that these petitions are pleasing to our Father in heaven, and are heard by Him; for He Himself has commanded us to pray in this way and has promised to hear us. Amen, amen means "yes, yes, it shall be so."

* These words were not in Luther's Small Catechism.

The Sacrament of Holy Baptism

As the head of the family should teach it in a simple way to his household

FIRST

What is Baptism?

Baptism is not just plain water, but it is the water included in God's command and combined with God's word.

Which is that word of God?

Christ our Lord says in the last chapter of Matthew: "Therefore go and make disciples of all nations, baptizing them in the name of the Father and of the Son and of the Holy Spirit." **(Matt. 28:19)**

SECOND

What benefits does Baptism give?

It works forgiveness of sins, rescues from death and the devil, and gives eternal salvation to all who believe this, as the words and promises of God declare.

Which are these words and promises of God?

Christ our Lord says in the last chapter of Mark: "Whoever believes and is baptized will be saved, but whoever does not believe will be condemned." **(Mark 16:16)**

THIRD

How can water do such great things?

Certainly not just water, but the word of God in and with the water does these things, along with the faith which trusts this word of God in the water. For without God's word the water is plain water and no Baptism. But with the word of God it is a Baptism, that is, a life-giving water, rich in grace, and a washing of the new birth in the Holy Spirit, as St. Paul says in Titus, chapter three:

"He saved us through the washing of rebirth and renewal by the Holy Spirit, whom He poured out on us generously through Jesus Christ our Savior, so that, having been justified by His grace, we might become heirs having the hope of eternal life. This is a trustworthy saying." **(Titus 3:5–8)**

FOURTH

What does such baptizing with water indicate?

It indicates that the Old Adam in us should by daily contrition and repentance be drowned and die with all sins and evil desires, and that a new man should daily emerge and arise to live before

God in righteousness and purity forever.

Where is this written?

St. Paul writes in Romans chapter six: "We were therefore buried with Him through baptism into death in order that, just as Christ was raised from the dead through the glory of the Father, we too may live a new life." **(Rom. 6:4)**

Confession

How Christians should be taught to confess

WHAT IS CONFESSION?

Confession has two parts.

First, that we confess our sins, and

second, that we receive absolution, that is, forgiveness, from the pastor as from God Himself, not doubting, but firmly believing that by it our sins are forgiven before God in heaven.

What sins should we confess?

Before God we should plead guilty of all sins, even those we are not aware of, as we do in the Lord's Prayer; but before the pastor we should confess only those sins which we know and feel in our hearts.

Which are these?

Consider your place in life according to the Ten Commandments: Are you a father, mother, son, daughter, husband, wife, or worker? Have you been disobedient, unfaithful, or lazy? Have you been hot-tempered, rude, or quarrelsome? Have you hurt someone by your words or deeds? Have you stolen, been negligent, wasted anything, or done any harm?

A Short Form of Confession

[Luther intended the following form to serve only as an example of private confession for Christians of his time. For a contemporary form of individual confession, see Lutheran Service Book, pp. 292–293.]

The penitent says:

Dear confessor, I ask you please to hear my confession and to pronounce forgiveness in order to fulfill God's will.

I, a poor sinner, plead guilty before God of all sins. In particular I confess before you that as a servant, maid, etc., I, sad to say, serve my master unfaithfully, for in this and that I have not done what I was told to do. I have made him angry and caused him to curse. I have been negligent and allowed damage to be done. I have also been offensive in words and deeds. I have quarreled with my peers. I have grumbled about the lady of the house and cursed her. I am sorry for all of this and I ask for grace. I want to do better.

A master or lady of the house may say:

In particular I confess before you that I have not faithfully guided my children, servants, and wife to the glory of God. I have cursed. I have set a bad example by indecent words and deeds. I have hurt my neighbor and spoken evil of him. I have overcharged, sold inferior merchandise, and given less than was paid for.

[Let the penitent confess whatever else he has done against God's commandments and his own position.]

If, however, someone does not find himself burdened with these or greater sins, he should not trouble himself or search for or invent other sins, and thereby make confession a torture. Instead, he should mention one or two that he knows: In particular I confess that I have cursed; I have used improper words; I have neglected this or that, etc. Let that be enough.

But if you know of none at all (which hardly seems possible), then mention none in particular, but receive the forgiveness upon the general confession which you make to God before the confessor.

Then the confessor shall say:

God be merciful to you and strengthen your faith. Amen.

Furthermore:

Do you believe that my forgiveness is God's forgiveness?

Yes, dear confessor.

Then let him, say:

Let it be done for you as you believe. And I, by the command of our Lord Jesus Christ, forgive you your sins in the name of the Father and of the Son and of the Holy Spirit. Amen. Go in peace.

A confessor will know additional passages with which to comfort and to strengthen the faith of those who have great burdens of conscience or are sorrowful and distressed.

This is intended only as a general form of confession.

WHAT IS THE OFFICE OF THE KEYS?*

The Office of the Keys is that special authority which Christ has given to His church on earth to forgive the sins of repentant sinners, but to withhold forgiveness from the unrepentant as long as they do not repent.

Where is this written?

This is what St. John the Evangelist writes in chapter twenty: The Lord Jesus breathed on His disciples and said, "Receive the Holy Spirit. If you forgive anyone his sins, they are forgiven; if you do not forgive them, they are not forgiven." (**John 20:22–23**)

What do you believe according to these words?

I believe that when the called ministers of Christ deal with us by His divine command, in particular when they exclude openly unrepentant sinners from the Christian congregation and absolve those who repent of their sins and want to do better, this is as valid and certain, even in heaven, as if Christ our dear Lord dealt with us Himself.

*This question may not have been composed by Luther himself but reflects his teaching and was included in editions of the catechism during his lifetime.

The Sacrament of the Altar

As the head of the family should teach it in a simple way to his household

What is the Sacrament of the Altar?

It is the true body and blood of our Lord Jesus Christ under the bread and wine, instituted by Christ Himself for us Christians to eat and to drink.

Where is this written?

The holy Evangelists Matthew, Mark, Luke, and St. Paul write:

Our Lord Jesus Christ, on the night when He was betrayed, took bread, and when He had given thanks, He broke it and gave it to the disciples and said: "Take, eat; this is My body, which is given for you. This do in remembrance of Me."

In the same way also He took the cup after supper, and when He had given thanks, He gave it to them, saying, "Drink of it, all of you; this cup is the new testament in My blood, which is shed for you for the forgiveness of sins. This do, as often as you drink it, in remembrance of Me."

What is the benefit of this eating and drinking?

These words, "Given and shed for you for the forgiveness of sins," show us that in the Sacrament forgiveness of sins, life, and salvation are given us through these words. For where there is forgiveness of sins, there is also life and salvation.

How can bodily eating and drinking do such great things?

Certainly not just eating and drinking do these things, but the words written here: "Given and shed for you for the forgiveness of sins." These words, along with the bodily eating and drinking, are the main thing in the Sacrament. Whoever believes these words has exactly what they say: "forgiveness of sins."

Who receives this sacrament worthily?

Fasting and bodily preparation are certainly fine outward training. But that person is truly worthy and well prepared who has faith in these words: "Given and shed for you for the forgiveness of sins."

But anyone who does not believe these words or doubts them is unworthy and unprepared, for the words "for you" require all hearts to believe.

SECTION 2
Daily Prayers

How the head of the family should teach his household to pray morning and evening

MORNING PRAYER

In the morning when you get up, make the sign of the holy cross and say:

In the name of the Father and of the † Son and of the Holy Spirit. Amen.

Then, kneeling or standing, repeat the Creed and the Lord's Prayer. If you choose, you may also say this little prayer:

I thank You, my heavenly Father, through Jesus Christ, Your dear Son, that You have kept me this night from all harm and danger; and I pray that You would keep me this day also from sin and every evil, that all my doings and life may please You. For into Your hands I commend myself, my body and soul, and all things. Let Your holy angel be with me, that the evil foe may have no power over me. Amen.

Then go joyfully to your work, singing a hymn, like that of the Ten Commandments, or whatever your devotion may suggest.

EVENING PRAYER

In the evening when you go to bed, make the sign of the holy cross and say:

In the name of the Father and of the † Son and of the Holy Spirit. Amen.

Then kneeling or standing, repeat the Creed and the Lord's Prayer. If you choose, you may also say this little prayer:

I thank You, my heavenly Father, through Jesus Christ, Your dear Son, that You have graciously kept me this day; and I pray that You would forgive me all my sins where I have done wrong, and graciously keep me this night. For into Your hands I commend myself, my body and soul, and all things. Let Your holy angel be with me, that the evil foe may have no power over me. Amen.

Then go to sleep at once and in good cheer.

How the head of the family should teach his household to ask a blessing and return thanks

ASKING A BLESSING

The children and members of the household shall go to the table reverently, fold their hands, and say:

The eyes of all look to You, [O Lord,] and You give them their food at the proper time. You open

Your hand and satisfy the desires of every living thing. (**Ps. 145:15–16**)

Then shall be said the Lord's Prayer and the following:

Lord God, heavenly Father, bless us and these Your gifts which we receive from Your bountiful goodness, through Jesus Christ, our Lord. Amen.

RETURNING THANKS

Also, after eating, they shall, in like manner, reverently and with folded hands say:

Give thanks to the Lord, for He is good. His love endures forever. [He] gives food to every creature. He provides food for the cattle and for the young ravens when they call. His pleasure is not in the strength of the horse, nor His delight in the legs of a man; the Lord delights in those who fear Him, who put their hope in His unfailing love. (**Ps. 136:1, 25; 147:9–11**)

Then shall be said the Lord's Prayer and the following:

We thank You, Lord God, heavenly Father, for all Your benefits, through Jesus Christ, our Lord, who lives and reigns with You and the Holy Spirit forever and ever. Amen.

SECTION 3
Table of Duties

Certain passages of Scripture for various holy orders and positions, admonishing them about their duties and responsibilities

To Bishops, Pastors, and Preachers

The overseer must be above reproach, the husband of but one wife, temperate, self-controlled, respectable, hospitable, able to teach, not given to drunkenness, not violent but gentle, not quarrelsome, not a lover of money. He must manage his own family well and see that his children obey him with proper respect. **1 Tim. 3:2–4**

He must not be a recent convert, or he may become conceited and fall under the same judgment as the devil. **1 Tim. 3:6**

He must hold firmly to the trustworthy message as it has been taught, so that he can encourage others by sound doctrine and refute those who oppose it. **Titus 1:9**

What the Hearers Owe Their Pastors

The Lord has commanded that those who preach the gospel should receive their living from the gospel. **1 Cor. 9:14**

Anyone who receives instruction in the word must share all good things with his instructor. Do not be deceived: God cannot be mocked. A man reaps what he sows. **Gal. 6:6–7**

The elders who direct the affairs of the church well are worthy of double honor, especially those whose work is preaching and teaching. For the Scripture says, "Do not muzzle the ox while it is treading out the grain," and "The worker deserves his wages." **1 Tim. 5:17–18**

We ask you, brothers, to respect those who work hard among you, who are over you in the Lord and who admonish you. Hold them in the highest regard in love because of their work. Live in peace with each other. **1 Thess. 5:12–13**

Obey your leaders and submit to their authority. They keep watch over you as men who must give an account. Obey them so that their work will be a joy, not a burden, for that would be of no advantage to you. **Heb. 13:17**

OF CIVIL GOVERNMENT

Everyone must submit himself to the governing authorities, for there is no authority except that which God has established. The authorities that exist have been established by God. Consequently, he who rebels against the authority is rebelling against what God has instituted, and those who do so will bring judgment on themselves. For rulers hold no terror for those who do right, but for those who do wrong. Do you want to be free from fear of the one in authority? Then do what is right and he will commend you. For he is God's servant to do you good. But if you do wrong, be afraid, for he does not bear the sword for nothing. He is God's servant, an agent of wrath to bring punishment on the wrongdoer. **Rom. 13:1–4**

OF CITIZENS

Give to Caesar what is Caesar's, and to God what is God's. **Matt. 22:21**

It is necessary to submit to the authorities, not only because of possible punishment but also because of conscience. This is also why you pay taxes, for the authorities are God's servants, who give their full time to governing. Give everyone what you owe him: If you owe taxes, pay taxes; if revenue, then revenue; if respect, then respect; if honor, then honor. **Rom. 13:5–7**

I urge, then, first of all, that requests, prayers, intercession and thanksgiving be made for everyone—for kings and all those in authority, that we may live peaceful and quiet lives, in all godliness and holiness. This is good, and pleases God our Savior. **1 Tim. 2:1–3**

Remind the people to be subject to rulers and authorities, to be obedient, to be ready to do whatever is good. **Titus 3:1**

Submit yourselves for the Lord's sake to every authority instituted among men: whether to the king, as the supreme authority, or to governors, who are sent by him to punish those who do wrong and to commend those who do right. **1 Peter 2:13–14**

To Husbands

Husbands, in the same way be considerate as you live with your wives, and treat them with respect as the weaker partner and as heirs with you of the gracious gift of life, so that nothing will hinder your prayers. **1 Peter 3:7**

Husbands, love your wives and do not be harsh with them. **Col. 3:19**

To Wives

Wives, submit to your husbands as to the Lord. **Eph. 5:22**

They were submissive to their own husbands, like Sarah, who obeyed Abraham and called him her master. You are her daughters if you do what is right and do not give way to fear. **1 Peter 3:5–6**

To Parents

Fathers, do not exasperate your children; instead, bring them up in the training and instruction of the Lord. **Eph. 6:4**

To Children

Children, obey your parents in the Lord, for this is right. "Honor your father and your mother" —which is the first commandment with a promise—"that it may go well with you and that you may enjoy long life on the earth." **Eph. 6:1–3**

To Workers of All Kinds

Slaves, obey your earthly masters with respect and fear, and with sincerity of heart, just as you would obey Christ. Obey them not only to win their favor when their eye is on you, but like slaves of Christ, doing the will of God from your heart. Serve wholeheartedly, as if you were serving the Lord, not men, because you know that the Lord will reward everyone for whatever good he does, whether he is slave or free. **Eph. 6:5–8**

To Employers and Supervisors

Masters, treat your slaves in the same way. Do not threaten them, since you know that He who is both their Master and yours is in heaven, and there is no favoritism with Him. **Eph. 6:9**

To Youth

Young men, in the same way be submissive to those who are older. All of you, clothe yourselves with humility toward one another, because, "God opposes the proud but gives grace to the humble." Humble yourselves, therefore, under God's mighty hand, that He may lift you up in due time. **1 Peter 5:5–6**

To Widows

The widow who is really in need and left all alone puts her hope in God and continues night and day to pray and to ask God for help. But the widow who lives for pleasure is dead even while she lives. **1 Tim. 5:5–6**

To Everyone

The commandments . . . are summed up in this one rule: "Love your neighbor as yourself." **Rom. 13:9**

I urge . . . that requests, prayers, intercession and thanksgiving be made for everyone. **1 Tim. 2:1**

Let each his lesson learn with care, and all the household well shall fare.

SECTION 4

Christian Questions with Their Answers *

Prepared by Dr. Martin Luther for those who intend to go to the Sacrament

After confession and instruction in the Ten Commandments, the Creed, the Lord's Prayer, and the Sacraments of Baptism and the Lord's Supper, the pastor may ask, or Christians may ask themselves these questions:

1. Do you believe that you are a sinner?
Yes, I believe it. I am a sinner.

* The "Christian Questions with Their Answers," designating Luther as the author, first appeared in an edition of the Small Catechism in 1551.

2. How do you know this?
From the Ten Commandments, which I have not kept.

3. Are you sorry for your sins?
Yes, I am sorry that I have sinned against God.

4. What have you deserved from God because of your sins?

His wrath and displeasure, temporal death, and eternal damnation. See **Rom. 6:21, 23.**

5. Do you hope to be saved?
Yes, that is my hope.

6. In whom then do you trust?
In my dear Lord Jesus Christ.

7. Who is Christ?
The Son of God, true God and man.

8. How many Gods are there?
Only one, but there are three persons: Father, Son, and Holy Spirit.

*9. What has Christ done for you that you
    trust in Him?*
He died for me and shed His blood for me on the cross for the forgiveness of sins.

10. Did the Father also die for you?
He did not. The Father is God only, as is the Holy Spirit; but the Son is both true God and true man. He died for me and shed His blood for me.

11. How do you know this?

From the holy Gospel, from the words instituting the Sacrament, and by His body and blood given me as a pledge in the Sacrament.

12. *What are the words of institution?*

Our Lord Jesus Christ, on the night when He was betrayed, took bread, and when He had given thanks, He broke it and gave it to the disciples and said: "Take eat; this is My body, which is given for you. This do in remembrance of Me."

In the same way also He took the cup after supper, and when He had given thanks, He gave it to them, saying: "Drink of it, all of you; this cup is the new testament in My blood, which is shed for you for the forgiveness of sins. This do, as often as you drink it, in remembrance of Me."

13. *Do you believe, then, that the true body and blood of Christ are in the Sacrament?*

Yes, I believe it.

14. *What convinces you to believe this?*

The word of Christ: Take, eat, this is My body; drink of it, all of you, this is My blood.

15. *What should we do when we eat His body and drink His blood, and in this way receive His pledge?*

We should remember and proclaim His death and the shedding of His blood, as He taught us: This do, as often as you drink it, in remembrance of Me.

16. Why should we remember and proclaim His death?

First, so we may learn to believe that no creature could make satisfaction for our sins. Only Christ, true God and man, could do that. Second, so we may learn to be horrified by our sins, and to regard them as very serious. Third, so we may find joy and comfort in Christ alone, and through faith in Him be saved.

17. What motivated Christ to die and make full payment for your sins?

His great love for His Father and for me and other sinners, as it is written in **John 14; Romans 5; Galatians 2;** and **Ephesians 5.**

18. Finally, why do you wish to go to the Sacrament?

That I may learn to believe that Christ, out of great love, died for my sin, and also learn from Him to love God and my neighbor.

19. What should admonish and encourage a Christian to receive the Sacrament frequently?

First, both the command and the promise of Christ the Lord. Second, his own pressing need, because of which the command, encouragement, and promise are given.

20. But what should you do if you are not aware of this need and have no hunger and thirst for the Sacrament?

To such a person no better advice can be given than this: first, he should touch his body to see if he still has flesh and blood. Then he should believe what the Scriptures say of it in **Galatians 5** and **Romans 7.**

Second, he should look around to see whether he is still in the world, and remember that there will be no lack of sin and trouble, as the Scriptures say in **John 15–16** and in **1 John 2** and **5.**

Third, he will certainly have the devil also around him, who with his lying and murdering day and night will let him have no peace, within or without, as the Scriptures picture him in **John 8** and **16; 1 Peter 5; Ephesians 6;** and **2 Timothy 2.**

NOTE

These questions and answers are no child's play, but are drawn up with great earnestness of purpose by the venerable and devout Dr. Luther for both young and old. Let each one pay attention and consider it a serious matter; for St. Paul writes to the Galatians in chapter six: "Do not be deceived: God cannot be mocked."

Index

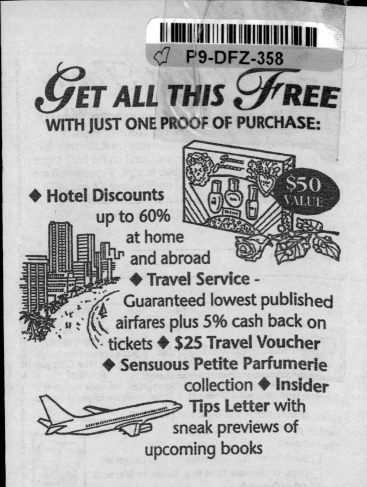

P9-DFZ-358

GET ALL THIS FREE

WITH JUST ONE PROOF OF PURCHASE:

$50 VALUE

◆ **Hotel Discounts** up to 60% at home and abroad ◆ **Travel Service** - Guaranteed lowest published airfares plus 5% cash back on tickets ◆ **$25 Travel Voucher** ◆ **Sensuous Petite Parfumerie** collection ◆ **Insider Tips Letter** with sneak previews of upcoming books

You'll get a FREE personal card, too. It's your passport to all these benefits— and to even more great gifts & benefits to come!

There's no club to join. No purchase commitment. No obligation.

HR-PP8A

Enrollment Form

☐ *Yes!* I WANT TO BE A *PRIVILEGED WOMAN*.
Enclosed is one *PAGES & PRIVILEGES*™ Proof of
Purchase from any Harlequin or Silhouette book currently for
sale in stores (Proofs of Purchase are found on the back pages
of books) and the store cash register receipt. Please enroll me
in *PAGES & PRIVILEGES*™. Send my Welcome Kit and FREE
Gifts – and activate my FREE benefits – immediately.

More great gifts and benefits to come.

NAME (please print)

ADDRESS   APT. NO

CITY   STATE   ZIP/POSTAL CODE

PROOF OF PURCHASE ONLY

**NO CLUB!
NO COMMITMENT!**
*Just one purchase brings
you great Free Gifts and
Benefits!*

Please allow 6-8 weeks for delivery. Quantities are limited. We reserve the right to
substitute items. Enroll before October 31, 1995 and receive one full year of benefits.

Name of store where this book was purchased_____

Date of purchase_____

Type of store:
☐ Bookstore   ☐ Supermarket   ☐ Drugstore
☐ Dept. or discount store (e.g. K-Mart or Walmart)
☐ Other (specify)_____

Which Harlequin or Silhouette series do you usually read?

_____

Complete and mail with one Proof of Purchase and store receipt to:
U.S.: *PAGES & PRIVILEGES*™, P.O. Box 1960, Danbury, CT 06813-1960
Canada: *PAGES & PRIVILEGES*™, 49-6A The Donway West, P.O. 813,
North York, ON M3C 2E8

HR-PP6B

▼ DETACH HERE AND MAIL TODAY! ▼

Dearest Reader,

Welcome to the town of Hard Luck, Alaska! I hope you'll join me there to meet the Midnight Sons, their families, friends and wives-to-be.

The people I want to credit with the idea for this project are, in fact, fictional—they're Valerie, Stephanie and Norah, the three sisters I wrote about in the *Orchard Valley* trilogy (Harlequin Romances #3232, #3239, #3244). I loved writing those books, I loved the characters and the town and last but definitely not least, I loved the way readers responded to the stories.

So when Harlequin suggested this six-book project, I was thrilled. Soon after that, the town of Hard Luck, the O'Halloran brothers and Midnight Sons all came to life. Never have I worked harder on a project, nor have I enjoyed my research more. In the summer of 1994, my husband and I traveled to Alaska, and I fell in love with the state—its sheer magnificence, the warmth of its people, the excitement of life on the "last frontier."

Now I invite you to sit back, put your feet up and allow me to introduce you to some proud, stubborn, *wonderful* men—Alaskan men—and show you what happens when they meet their real matches. Women from the "lower forty-eight." Women with the courage to change their lives and take risks for love. Women a lot like you and me!

Love,

Debbie

Debbie Macomber is one of the most popular romance authors writing today. She's written more than seventy romances (for Harlequin and Silhouette) and several bestselling "mainstream" women's fiction novels. Not surprisingly, Debbie has won a number of awards for her books.

She lives in Washington State with her husband, Wayne, and their dog, Peterkins. They have four grown children—and they've just become grandparents! Debbie's *thrilled* with her new granddaughter, Jazmine Lynn.

Debbie loves to hear from readers. You can reach her at: P.O. Box 1458, Port Orchard, Washington 98366.

Books by Debbie Macomber

HARLEQUIN ROMANCE

Midnight Sons is a six-book series. The titles are:

Don't miss any of our special offers. Write to us at the following address for information on our newest releases.

Harlequin Reader Service
U.S.: 3010 Walden Ave., P.O. Box 1325, Buffalo, NY 14269
Canadian: P.O. Box 609, Fort Erie, Ont. L2A 5X3

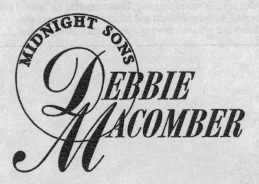

MIDNIGHT SONS

DEBBIE MACOMBER

Brides for Brothers

Harlequin Books

TORONTO • NEW YORK • LONDON
AMSTERDAM • PARIS • SYDNEY • HAMBURG
STOCKHOLM • ATHENS • TOKYO • MILAN
MADRID • WARSAW • BUDAPEST • AUCKLAND

ISBN 0-373-03379-6

BRIDES FOR BROTHERS

First North American Publication 1995.

Copyright © 1995 by Debbie Macomber.

Printed in U.S.A.

The History of Hard Luck, Alaska

Hard Luck, situated fifty miles north of the Arctic Circle, near the Brooks Range, was founded by Adam O'Halloran and his wife, Anna, in 1931. Adam came to Alaska to make his fortune, but never found the gold strike he sought. Nevertheless, the O'Hallorans and their two young sons, Charles and David, stayed on—in part because of a tragedy that befell the family a few years later.

Other prospectors and adventurers began to move to Hard Luck, some of them bringing wives and children. The town became a stopping-off place for mail, equipment and supplies. The Fletcher family arrived in 1938 to open a dry goods store.

When World War II began, Hard Luck's population was fifty or sixty people, all told. Some of the young men, including the O'Halloran sons, joined the armed services; Charles left for Europe in 1942, David in 1944 at the age of eighteen. Charles died during the fighting. Only David came home—with a young English war bride, Ellen Sawyer (despite the fact that he'd become engaged to Catherine Fletcher shortly before going overseas).

After the war, David qualified as a bush pilot. He then built some small cabins to attract the sport fisherman and hunters who were starting to come to Alaska; he also worked as a guide. Eventually, in the early seventies, he built a lodge to replace the cabins—a lodge that later burned to the ground.

David and Ellen had three sons, born fairly late in their marriage—Charles (named after David's brother) was born in 1960, Sawyer in 1963 and Christian in 1965.

Hard Luck had been growing slowly all this time, and by 1970 it was home to just over a hundred people. These were the years of the oil boom, when the school and community center were built by the state. After Vietnam, ex-serviceman Ben Hamilton joined the community and opened the Hard Luck Café, which became the social focus for the town.

In the late 1980s, the three O'Halloran brothers formed a partnership, creating Midnight Sons, a bush-pilot operation. They were awarded the mail contract, and also deliver fuel and other necessities to the interior. In addition, they serve as a small commuter airline, flying passengers to and from Fairbanks and within the North Arctic.

At the time these stories start, there are approximately 150 people living in Hard Luck—a preponderance of them male....

PROLOGUE

"WHAT YOU REALLY NEED are *women*."

Sawyer O'Halloran made a show of choking on his coffee. "Women! We've got enough problems!"

Ben Hamilton—the Hard Luck Café's owner, cook and just about everything else—set the coffeepot down on the counter. "Didn't you just tell me Phil Duncan's decided to move back to Fairbanks?"

Phil was the best pilot Sawyer had. He wasn't the first one Midnight Sons had lost to the big city, either. Every time a pilot resigned, it was a setback for the Arctic flight service.

"Yes, but Phil's not leaving because of a woman," Sawyer muttered.

"Sure he is," Duke Porter piped up. Still clutching his mug, he slipped onto the stool next to Sawyer. "Phil quit because he couldn't see his girlfriend as much as he wanted, and everyone knows it. He might've given you some phony excuse when he handed in his notice, but you know as well as I do why he decided to quit."

"Joe and Harlan left because of women, too. Because they couldn't meet any living here!" It was Ben again. The ex-Navy 'stew burner'—as the O'Halloran brothers called him—obviously had strong opinions on this issue. Sawyer often shared his opinion, but not this time. He had half a mind to suggest Ben keep his nose out of this, but that wouldn't be fair.

One of the problems with living in a small town was that you'd known most of the people all your life, Sawyer reflected. Everyone knew your damn business.

He might as well set up the Midnight Sons office right here in the middle of the café. His pilots routinely ate breakfast at Ben's, and the cook was as familiar with the air charter's troubles as the brothers were themselves.

Christian, the youngest O'Halloran, cupped his mug with both hands. "All right, if you won't say it, I will," he began, looking pointedly at Sawyer. "Ben's right. Bringing a few women to Hard Luck would keep the crew happy."

Sawyer didn't really disagree with him. "We've got a new schoolteacher coming. A woman." As a member of the school board, Sawyer had read over Bethany Ross's application and been impressed with her qualifications, but he wasn't sure the state should have hired her. She'd been born and raised in California. He still hadn't figured out why she'd applied for a teaching position north of the Arctic Circle.

"I just hope this teacher isn't like the last one," John Henderson grumbled. "I flew her in, remember? I was as polite as could be, circled the area a bit, showed her the sights from the air, talked up the town. I'll be damned, but the woman wouldn't even get off the plane."

"I'd still like to know what you said to her," Christian muttered.

"I didn't say anything," John insisted. "Besides, the new teacher's not coming until August, is she?"

"August," Ben repeated. "*One* woman." He readjusted his stained white apron around his thick waist. "I can see it all now."

"See what?" Fool that he was, Sawyer had to ask. It went without saying that Ben would be more than happy to tell him.

"One woman will cause more problems than she'll alleviate," Ben said in a portentous voice. "Think about it, Sawyer."

Sawyer didn't want to think about it. All this talk of bringing in women made him uncomfortable. In his opinion, it was asking for trouble.

"One thing's for sure, we aren't going to let John fly her in this time," Ralph said scornfully. "I got first dibs."

He was answered by a loud chorus of "Like hell!" and "No way!"

"Don't squabble!" Sawyer shouted.

Ben chuckled and slid a plate of sourdough hotcakes onto the counter toward Ralph.

"See what I mean?" the cook said under his breath. "Your men are already fighting over the new teacher, and she isn't even arriving for months."

Ralph lit into the hotcakes as if he hadn't eaten in a week. Mouth full, he mumbled something about lonely bachelors.

"All right, all right," Sawyer conceded. "Bringing a few women to Hard Luck just might be a good idea, but how do you propose we persuade them to move up here?"

"I guess we could advertise," Christian said thoughtfully, then brightened. "Sure, we'll advertise. It's a hell of a good idea. I don't know why we didn't think of it sooner."

"Advertise?" Sawyer glared at his brother. "What do you mean, *advertise?*"

"Well, we could put an ad in one of those glossy magazines women like to buy. What I heard, it's gotten to be the ' in thing to place an ad about lonely men in Alaska seeking companionship."

"A friend of a friend sent his picture to one of those," Ralph said excitedly, "and before he knew it, he had a sackful of letters. All from women eager to meet him."

"I want you to know right now I'm not taking off my shirt and posing for any damn picture," Duke Porter said in an emphatic voice.

"Getting your photograph in one of those magazine isn't as easy as it sounds," Ralph warned after swallowing a huge bite. He stiffened his shoulders. "Not that I've tried or anything."

"Things are rarely as good as they sound," Sawyer pointed out reasonably, pleased that at least one of his employees was thinking clearly.

"Those women aren't looking for pen pals, you know," John muttered. "They're after husbands, and they aren't the kind who can be picky, either, if you catch my drift."

"So? You guys aren't exactly centerfold material yourselves," Ben was quick to remind them. He pushed up the sleeves of his shirt and planted his hands on the counter.

"As far as I can see," Sawyer said, "we don't have anything to offer women. It isn't likely our good looks would induce them to move here, now is it?"

John's face fell with disappointment. "You're probably right."

"What would work, then?" Christian asked. "We need to think positive, or we're going to end up spending our lives alone."

"I don't have any complaints about *my* life," Sawyer told his brother. Christian's enthusiasm for this crazy idea surprised him. Sawyer was willing to go along with it, but he didn't have much faith in its success. For one thing, he was afraid the presence of these new women might well create a whole set of new problems. Besides, his men had a snowball's chance in hell of luring women to Hard Luck. At least none who'd stay more than a few weeks.

"You've got to remember women aren't that different from men," Christian was saying, sounding like a TV talk-show expert.

The others stared at him, and Christian laughed. "You know what I mean. You guys came up to Hard Luck, despite the fact that we're fifty miles north of the Arctic Circle."

"Sure," Duke answered. "But the wages are the best around, and the living conditions aren't bad."

"Wages," Christian said, reaching for a pen in the pocket of his plaid shirt. He made a note on his paper napkin.

"You aren't thinking about *paying* women to move to Hard Luck, are you?" Sawyer would fight that idea tooth and nail. He'd be damned if he'd see his hard-earned cash wasted on such foolishness.

"We could offer women jobs, couldn't we?" Christian asked. He looked around to gather support from the other pilots.

"Doing what?" Sawyer demanded.

"Well . . ." Frowning, his brother gnawed on the end of his pen. "You've been saying for a long time that we need to get the office organized. How about hiring a secretary? You and I have enough to do dealing with everything else. It's a mess, and we can't seem to get ahead."

Sawyer resisted the urge to suggest a correspondence course on time management. "All right," he said grudgingly.

The other pilots looked up from their breakfasts. They were beginning to take notice.

"What about all those books your mother left for Hard Luck after she married Frank?" Ben asked. "It seems to me there was some talk about starting up a library."

Sawyer gritted his teeth. "A volunteer library."

"But someone's got to organize it," Christian said. "I've tried now and again, but every time I even start to get things straightened out, I'm overwhelmed. There must be a thousand books there."

Sawyer couldn't really object, since, unlike Christian, he'd never made any effort to put his mother's vast collection in order.

"That was a generous thing your mother did, giving the town her books," Ralph said. "But it's a damn shame we can't find what we want or check it out if we do."

"It seems to me," Christian said, smiling broadly, "that we could afford to pay someone to set up the library and run it for a year or so, see how it works. Don't you agree?"

Sawyer shrugged. "If Charles does." But they both knew their oldest brother would endorse the idea. He'd been wanting to get the library going for quite a while.

"I heard Pearl say she was thinking of moving to Nenana to live with her daughter," Ben told the gathering. "In that case, the town's going to need someone with medical experience for the health clinic."

A number of heads nodded. Sawyer suspected now was not the time to remind everyone that Pearl routinely mentioned moving in with her daughter. Generally the sixty-year-old woman came up with the idea in the darkest part of winter, when there were only a couple of hours of daylight and spirits were low.

"I know what you're thinking," Ben said, glancing at Sawyer. "But did you ever stop to think that Pearl actually *would* leave if someone was here to take over for her?"

No, Sawyer hadn't. Pearl had lived in Hard Luck for as long as he could remember. She'd been a friend to his mother when Ellen had lived in Hard Luck, and a peacemaker in the small community. Over the years Sawyer had frequently had opportunity to be grateful to Pearl. If she did decide to move, he'd miss her.

"We can ask her if she's serious about wanting to retire," Sawyer agreed, despite the reluctance. "But I won't have Pearl thinking we don't want her."

"I'll talk to her myself," Christian promised.

"I could use a bit of help around here," Ben said. "I've been feeling my age of late."

"You mean feeling your oats, don't you?" John teased.

Ben grinned. "Go ahead and add a part-time cook and waitress to your list."

There were smiles all around. Sawyer hated to be the one to put a damper on all these plans, but someone had to open their eyes to a few truths. "Has anyone figured out where these women are going to live?"

It was almost comical to see the smiles fall in unison, as if a puppetmaster were working their mouths. Though Sawyer had to admit he was beginning to warm to the idea of recruiting women. Hard Luck could do with a few new faces and he wouldn't object if those faces happened to be young, female and pretty. Not that *he* was the marrying kind. No, sirree. Not Sawyer O'Halloran. Not after what he'd seen with his parents. Their unhappiness had taught him early and taught him well that marriage meant misery. Although, in his opinion, Catherine Fletcher bore a lot of the blame there. . . .

He shook his head. Marriage was definitely out, and he suspected his two brothers felt the same way. They must. Neither of them seemed inclined toward marriage. It was just as well.

He returned his attention to the dilemma at hand. No one appeared to have any answers about where these women would live, and Sawyer felt obligated to point out the less-than-favorable aspects of their plan. The more he considered, the more certain he became that this idea was impossible. Attractive, perhaps—especially in a moment of weakness—but impossible.

"It wouldn't have worked, anyway," he said.

"Why not?" The question came from his brother.

"Women are never satisfied with the status quo. They'd move to Hard Luck and immediately want to change things." Sawyer had seen it before. "Well, *I* don't want things changed. We have it good here—damn good."

"You're right," Ralph agreed, but without any real enthusiasm.

"Before we knew how it happened," Sawyer continued, "the ladies would have rings on their fingers and through our noses, they'd be leading us around like . . . like sheep. Worse, they'd convince us that was just the way we wanted it."

"Nope. Not going to happen to me," John vowed. "Unless . . ."

Not giving him a chance to weaken, Sawyer went on. "Before we knew it, we'd be making runs into Fairbanks for low-fat ice cream because one or another of them has a craving for chocolate without the calories." Sawyer could picture it now. "They'd want us to watch our language and turn the TV off during dinner and shave every day...and..."

"You're right," Duke said with conviction. "A woman would probably want me to shave off my beard."

The men grimaced as if they could already feel the razor cut across their skin.

Women in Hard Luck would have his pilots wrapped around their little fingers within a week, Sawyer thought. Following that, his men wouldn't be worth a damn.

Christian hadn't spoken for several moments. Now he slowly rubbed his hand along the underside of his jaw. "What about the cabins?"

"The old hunting cabins your father built on the outskirts of town?" Ralph asked.

Sawyer and Christian exchanged looks. "Those are the ones," Christian said. "Dad built them back in the fifties before the lodge was completed—you know, the lodge that burned? Folks would fly in for hunting and fishing and he'd put them up there. They're simple, one medium-size room without any of the conveniences."

"No one's lived in those cabins for years," Sawyer reminded his brother.

"But they're solid, and other than a little dirt there's nothing wrong with them. Someone could live there. Easily." Christian's voice rose as he grew excited about the idea. "With a little soap and water and a few minor repairs, they'd be livable in nothing flat."

Sawyer couldn't believe what he was hearing. A city gal would take one look at those cabins and leave on the next flight out. "But there isn't any running water or electricity."

"No," Christian agreed, "not yet."

Now Sawyer understood, and he didn't like it. "I'm not putting any money into fixing up those run-down shacks." Charles would have a fit if he let Christian talk him into doing anything so stupid.

"Those old cabins aren't worth much, are they?" Christian asked.

Sawyer hesitated. He recognized his brother's tone. Christian had something up his sleeve.

"No," Sawyer admitted cautiously.

"Then it wouldn't hurt to give the cabins away."

"Give them away?" Sawyer repeated. It stood to reason that no one would *pay* for them. Who'd want them, even if they were free?

"We're going to need something to induce women to move to Hard Luck, don't you think?" Christian asked. "We aren't offering them marriage."

"You're damn right we're not," John said.

"Companionship is all I'm interested in," another one of the pilots added. "Female companionship."

"We don't want to mislead anyone into thinking we're offering marriage."

"Exactly."

"I'm not the marrying kind."

Sawyer looked around the room at his pilots. "Marriage is what most women are after," he said with more certainty than he actually felt.

"There's plenty of jobs in the lower forty-eight," Christian said, sounding perfectly logical. This was generally where Sawyer ran into trouble when it came to dealing with his younger brother. Christian could propose the most ridiculous idea in the most methodical, reasonable way. "True?"

"True," Sawyer agreed warily.

"Then, like I said before, we've got to give these women some incentive to live and work in Hard Luck."

"You want to give them the cabins?" Sawyer scratched the side of his head. "As an *incentive?*"

"Sure. Then if they want to add electricity and running water they can do it with their own money."

Sawyer checked around to see what the others were thinking. He couldn't find a dissenting look among them. Not on Ben's face and certainly not on any of the others. He should have known Christian's idea would quickly take root in the fertile minds of his women-starved men.

"We'd clean the cabins up a bit first," Christian said as though this was the least they could do.

"We found a bear in one of them last year," Sawyer reminded his brother.

"That bear didn't mean any harm," Ralph said confidently. "He was just getting a good look around, is all. I doubt he'll be back after the shot of pepper spray Mitch gave him."

Sawyer just shook his head, bemused.

"But it might not be a good idea to mention the bear to any of the women," Ben was quick to add. "Women are funny about wild critters."

"Yeah," John added in hushed tones, "take my word for it—don't say anything about the wildlife."

"Say anything?" Sawyer asked. The men made it sound like he was going to personally interview each applicant.

"To the women when you talk to them," Ralph explained with exaggerated patience.

"I'm going to be talking to these women?"

"Why, sure," Duke said, as if that had been understood from the beginning. "You'll have to interview them, you or Christian. Especially if you're going to offer them housing when they accept a job in Hard Luck."

"You'd better throw in some land while you're at it," Ben said, reaching for the coffeepot. He refilled the mugs and set the pot back on the burner. "You O'Hallorans got far more of it than you know what to do with. Offer the women a cabin and twenty acres of land if they'll live and work in Hard Luck for one year."

"Great idea."

"Just like the good old days when the settlers first arrived."

"Those cabins aren't *on* any twenty acres." Sawyer raised his arms to stop the discussion. "It'd be misleading to let anyone think they were, or that—"

"No one said the cabins had to be on acreage, did they?" Duke broke in. "Besides, to my way of thinking, people shouldn't look a gift house in the mouth." He chuckled at his own feeble joke.

"A year sounds fair," Christian said decisively, ignoring him. "If it doesn't work out, then they're free to leave, no hard feelings."

"No hard feelings," John echoed.

"Now, just a minute," Sawyer said. Was he the only one who possessed a lick of sense? He'd come into the Hard Luck Café for a simple cup of coffee, discouraged by the news that Phil was leaving. The morning had quickly gone from bad to worse.

"How are we going to let women know about your offer?" Ralph asked.

"We'll take out ads just the way we first said," Christian told him. "I've got a business trip planned to Seattle, and I'll interview the women who apply."

"Hold your horses," Sawyer said, frowning. "We can't go giving away those cabins, never mind the acreage, without discussing it with Charles first. Besides, there are anti-discrimination laws that make it impossible to advertise a job for women only."

Christian grinned. "There're ways around that."

Sawyer rolled his eyes. "But we really need to discuss this with Charles." Their oldest brother was a silent partner in the O'Hallorans' air charter service. He should have a voice in this decision; after all, they'd be offering family-owned cabins and land.

"There isn't time for that," Christian argued. "Charles'll go along with it. You know he will. He hasn't paid that much attention to the business since he started working for Alaska Oil."

"You'd better have an attorney draw up some kind of contract," Ben suggested.

"Right." Christian added that to his list. "I'll get on it right away. Magazines take too long, but I'll write the ad this morning and see about getting it in the Seattle paper. It might be best if we placed it in another city, as well. It wouldn't be much trouble to drive down to Oregon and interview women from Portland. I've got plenty of time."

"Sounds like a good idea."

"I'll make up the application form," Sawyer offered reluctantly. This was happening much too fast. "You know, guys . . ." He hated to be the one to throw another wrench in the works, but someone needed a clear head, and it was obvious he'd been elected. "If any woman's foolish enough to respond, those old cabins had better be in decent shape. It's going to take a lot of work."

"I'll help," John said enthusiastically.

"Me, too."

"I expect we all will." Duke drained the last of his coffee, then narrowed his gaze on Christian. "Just make sure you get a blonde for me."

"A blonde," Christian repeated.

Sawyer closed his eyes and groaned. He had a bad feeling about all this. A very bad feeling.

CHAPTER ONE

IT HAD BEEN one of those days. Abbey Sutherland made herself a cup of tea, then sat in the large overstuffed chair and propped her feet on the ottoman. She closed her eyes, soaking in the silence.

The morning had started badly when Scott overslept, which had caused him and Susan to miss the school bus. Seven-year-old Susan had insisted on wearing her pink sweater, which was still in the dirty-clothes hamper, and she'd whined all the way to school. Abbey had driven them, catching every red light en route.

By the time she arrived at the library, she was ten minutes late. Mrs. Duffy tossed her a look that could have curdled milk.

But those minor irritations faded after lunch. Abbey received notice that the library's budget for the next fiscal year had been reduced and two positions would be cut—the positions held by the most recently hired employees. In other words, Abbey was going to lose her job in less than three months.

She finally got home at six o'clock, tired, short-tempered and depressed. That was when Mr. Erickson, the manager of the apartment complex, hand-delivered the note informing her the rents were being raised.

It was the kind of day even hot fudge couldn't cover.

Sensing her mood, the kids had acted up all evening. Abbey was exhausted, and she didn't think reruns of "Matlock" were going to help.

Sipping her tea, she wondered what had happened to set her life off course this way. She had a savings account, but there wasn't enough in it to pay more than a month's worth of bills. She refused to go to her parents for money. Not again. It had been too humiliating the first time, although they'd been eager to help. Not once had her mother or father said "I told you so," but they'd issued plenty of warnings when she'd announced her intention to marry Dick Sutherland. They'd been right. Five years and two children later, Abbey had returned to Seattle emotionally battered, broken-hearted. And just plain broke.

Her parents had helped her back on her feet despite their limited income and lent her the money to finish her education. Abbey had painstakingly repaid every penny, but it had taken her almost three years.

The newspaper, still rolled up, lay at her feet, and she reached for it. She might as well start reading through the want ads now, though she wasn't likely to find another job as an assistant librarian. With cuts in local government spending, positions in libraries were becoming rare these days. But if she was willing to relocate...

"Mom." Scott stood beside her chair.

"Yes." She climbed out of her depression long enough to manage a smile for her nine-year-old son.

"Jason's dog had puppies."

Abbey felt her chest tighten. Scott had been asking for a dog all year. "Honey, we've already been over this a hundred times. The apartment complex doesn't allow pets."

"I didn't say I wanted one," he said defensively. "All I said was that Jason's dog had puppies. I know I can't have a dog as long as we live here, but I was just thinking that maybe with the rent increase we might move.''

"And if we do move," Abbey said, "you want me to look for a place where we can have a dog."

Her son grinned broadly. "Jason's puppies are really, really cute, Mom. You know what kind are my favorite?"

She did, but she played along. "Tell me."

"Huskies."

"Because the University of Washington mascot is a husky."

"Sort of, but they have cool eyes, don't they? And I really like the way their tails loop up. I know they're too big for me to have as a house pet, but I still like them best."

Abbey held out her arm to her son. He didn't cuddle with her much anymore. That was kid stuff to a boy who was almost ten. But tonight he seemed willing to forget that.

He clambered into the chair next to her, rested his head against her shoulder and sighed expressively. "I'm sorry I overslept this morning," he whispered.

"I'm sorry I yelled at you."

"That's all right. I figured I had it coming. I promise to get out of bed when you call from now on, okay?"

"Okay." Abbey closed her eyes, breathing in the clean shampoo scent of his hair.

They sat together a few minutes longer, saying nothing.

"You better get back to bed," Abbey said, although she was reluctant to see him go.

Scott climbed out of the chair. "Are we going to move?" he asked, looking at her with wide-eyed expectancy.

"I guess we will," she said, and smiled.

"'Night, Mom." Scott smiled, too, then turned and walked down the hall to his bedroom.

Abbey's heart felt a little lighter as she picked up the paper and peeled away the rubber band. She didn't bother to look at the front page, but turned directly to the classifieds.

The square box with the large block printing attracted her attention almost immediately. "LONELY MEN IN HARD LUCK, ALASKA, OFFER JOBS, HOMES AND LAND." Below in smaller print was a list of the positions open.

Abbey's heart stopped when she saw "librarian."

Hard Luck, Alaska. Jobs. A home with land. Twenty acres. Good grief, that was more than her grandfather had owned when he grew raspberries in Puyallup a generation earlier.

Dragging out an atlas, Abbey flipped through the pages until she found Alaska. Her finger ran down the list of town names until she found Hard Luck. Population 150.

She swallowed. A small town generally meant a sense of community. That excited her. As a girl, she'd spent summers on her grandparents' farm and loved it. She wanted to give her children the same opportunity. She was sure the three of them could adjust to life in a small town. In Alaska.

Using the atlas's directions to locate the town, Abbey drew her finger across one side of the page and down the other.

Her excitement died. Hard Luck was above the Arctic Circle. Oh, my. In that case, it probably *wasn't* such a great idea.

THE FOLLOWING MORNING, Abbey reviewed her options.

She set out a box of cold cereal, along with a carton of milk. A still-sleepy Scott and Susan pulled out chairs and sat at the table.

"Kids," she said, drawing a deep breath, "what would you say if I suggested we move to Alaska?"

"Alaska?" Scott perked up right away. "That's where they raise huskies!"

"Yes, I know."

"It's cold there, isn't it?" Susan asked.

"Real cold. Probably colder than it's ever been in Seattle."

"Colder than Texas?"

"Lots colder," Scott said with the superior older-brother tone. "It's so cold you don't even need refrigerators, isn't that right, Mom?"

"Uh, I think they probably still use them."

"But they wouldn't need to if they didn't have electricity. Right?"

"Right."

"Could I have a dog there?"

Abbey weighed her answer carefully. "We'd have to find that out after we arrived."

"Would Grandma and Grandpa come and visit?" Susan asked.

"I'm sure they would, and if they didn't, we could visit them."

Scott poured cereal into his bowl until it threatened to spill over.

"I read an ad in the paper last night. Hard Luck, Alaska, needs a librarian, and it looks like I'm going to need a new job soon."

Scott and Susan didn't comment.

"I didn't think it would be fair to call and ask for an interview without discussing it with both of you first."

"I think you should go for it," Scott advised, but Abbey could see visions of huskies in her son's bright blue eyes.

"It'll mean a big change for all of us."

"Is there snow there all the time?" Susan wanted to know.

"I don't think so, but I'll ask." Abbey hesitated, wondering exactly how much she should tell her children. "The ad said that the job comes with a cabin and twenty acres of land."

The spoon was poised in front of Scotty's mouth. "To keep?"

Abbey nodded. "But we'd need to live there for a year. I imagine there won't be many applicants, but then I don't know. There doesn't seem to be an abundance of jobs for assistant librarians, either."

"I could live anywhere for a year. Go for it, Mom!"

"Susan?" Abbey suspected the decision would be more difficult for her daughter.

"Will there be girls my age?"

"I don't know. Probably, but I can't guarantee that. The town only has 150 people, and it would be very different from the life we have here in Seattle."

"Come on, Susan," Scott urged. "We could have our very own house."

Susan's small shoulders heaved in a great sigh. "Do you want to move, Mommy?"

Abbey brushed the thick brown hair from her daughter's forehead. Call her greedy. Call her materialistic. Call her a sucker, but she couldn't stop thinking about those twenty acres and that cabin. No mortgage. Land. Security. And a job she loved. All in Hard Luck, Alaska.

She inhaled deeply, then nodded.

"Then I guess it would be all right."

Scott let out a holler and leapt from his chair. He grabbed Abbey's hands and danced them around the room.

"I haven't got the job yet," Abbey cried, breathless.

"But you'll get it," Scott said confidently.

Abbey sincerely hoped her son was right.

CHAPTER TWO

ABBEY TOOK several calming breaths before walking up to the hotel desk and giving her name.

"Mr. O'Halloran's taking interviews in the Snoqualamie Room on the second floor," the clerk told her.

Abbey's fingers tightened around her résumé as she headed for the escalator. Her heart pounded heavily, feeling like a lead weight in her chest.

Her decision to apply for this position had understandably received mixed reactions. Both Scott and Susan were excited about the prospect of a new life in Hard Luck, but Abbey's parents were hesitant.

Marie Murray would miss spoiling her grandchildren. Abbey's father, Wayne, was convinced she didn't know what she was getting into moving to the frozen north. But he seemed to forget that she made her living in a library. Soon after placing the initial call, Abbey had checked out a number of excellent books depicting life in Alaska. Her research had told her everything she wanted to know—and more.

Nevertheless, she'd already decided to accept the job, if it was offered. Living in Hard Luck would be better than having to accept money from her parents, no matter how cold the winters were.

Abbey found the Snoqualamie Room easily enough and glanced inside. A lean, rawboned man in his early thirties sat at a table reading intently. The hotel staff must have thought applicants would arrive thirsty, because they'd supplied a pitcher of ice water and at least two dozen glasses.

"Hello," she said with an expectant smile. "I'm Abbey Sutherland."

"Abbey." The man stood abruptly as if she'd caught him unawares. "I'm Christian O'Halloran. We spoke on the phone." He motioned to the seat on the other side of the table. "Make yourself comfortable."

She sat and handed him her résumé.

He barely glanced at it before setting it aside. "Thank you. I'll read it over later."

Abbey nervously folded her hands in her lap and waited.

"You're applying for the position of librarian, right?"

"Yes. I'm working toward my degree in library science."

"In other words you're not a full librarian."

"That's correct. In Washington state, a librarian is required to have a master's degree in library science. For the last two years I've worked as a librarian assistant for King County." She paused. Christian O'Halloran was difficult to read. "As an assistant librarian I answer reference questions, do quick information retrieval and customer service, and I have computer skills." She hesitated, wondering if she should continue.

"That sounds perfect. Hard Luck doesn't exactly have a library at the present moment. We do have a building, of sorts..."

"Books?"

"Oh, yes, hundreds of those. They were a gift to the town, and we need someone who's capable of handling every aspect of organizing a lending library."

"I'd be fully capable of that." She listed a number of responsibilities she'd handled in her job with the King County library system. Somehow, though, Abbey couldn't shake the feeling that Christian O'Halloran wasn't really interested in hearing about her qualifications.

He mentioned the pay, and although it wasn't as much as she was earning with King County, she wouldn't need to worry about paying rent.

A short silence followed, almost as if he wasn't sure what else to ask.

"Could you tell me a little about the library building?"

"Oh, sure. Actually it was a home at one time—my grandfather's original homestead, in fact—but I don't think you'd have much of a problem turning it into a usable library, would you?"

"Probably not."

Already, Abbey's mind was at work, dividing up the house. One of the bedrooms could be used for fiction, another for nonfiction. The dining room would be perfect for a reading room, or it could be set up as an area for children.

"You understand that life in Hard Luck isn't going to be anything like Seattle," Christian commented, breaking into her thoughts.

Her father had said that very thing the day before. "I realize that. Would you mind if I asked you about the house and the land you're offering?"

"Not at all."

"Well, uh, could you tell me about the house?"

She waited.

"Actually it's a cabin, and I'd describe it as...rustic." He seemed to stumble on the word. "It definitely has a...rural feel. Don't get me wrong, it's comfortable, but it's different from what you're used to."

"I'm sure it is. Tell me something about Hard Luck."

The man across from her relaxed. "It's probably the most beautiful place on earth. You might think I'm prejudiced and I can't very well deny it. I guess you'll have to form your own opinion.

"In summer there's sunlight nearly twenty-four hours a day. That's when the wildflowers bloom. I swear every color under the sun bursts to life, almost overnight. The forests and tundra turn scarlet and gold and burnt orange."

"It sounds lovely." And it did. "What about the winters?"

"Oh, yes, well, again it's beautiful, but the beauty is more fragile. I don't think anyone's really lived until they've viewed our light show."

"The aurora borealis."

"I'm not going to lie to you," Christian continued. "It gets mighty cold. In winter it isn't uncommon to have the temperature drop to forty or fifty below."

"My goodness." Although Abbey knew this, hearing him say it reinforced the reality.

"On those days, almost everything closes down. We don't generally fly when it's that cold. It's too hard on the planes, and even harder on the pilots."

Abbey nodded. He'd told her about Midnight Sons, the O'Halloran brothers' air charter service, during their telephone conversation.

"What about everything else?" she asked. "Like the school." He'd also explained in their previous conversation that Hard Luck had a school that went from kindergarten to twelfth grade.

"Life in town comes to a standstill, and we all kind of snuggle together. There's nothing to do in weather that cold but wait it out. Most days, we manage to keep the school open, though." He paused. "We rely on one another in Hard Luck. We have to."

"What about food?"

"We've got a grocery. It's not a supermarket, mind you, but it carries the essentials. Everyone in town stocks up on supplies once a year. But if you run out of anything, there's always the grocery. If Pete Livengood—he's the guy who owns the grocery—if he doesn't have what you need, one of the pilots can pick it up for you. Midnight Sons makes daily flights into Fairbanks. Oil's delivered once a day, so it isn't like you're stuck there."

"What about driving to Fairbanks? When I looked up Hard Luck in the atlas, I couldn't make out any roads. There is one, isn't there?"

"Sure there is—in a manner of speaking," Christian said proudly. "We got ourselves a haul road a few years back."

Abbey was relieved. If she did get the job, she'd have to have her furniture and other household effects delivered; without a road, that would have been a problem. Flying them was sure to be prohibitively expensive.

"Do you have any more questions for me?" she asked.

"None." Christian looked at his watch. "Would you mind filling out the application form while you're here? I'll be holding interviews for the next day or so. I'll give you a call tomorrow afternoon, if that's all right."

Abbey stood. "That'd be fine."

Christian handed her the one-page application, which she completed quickly and handed back to him.

He rose from behind the table and extended his hand. "It was a pleasure to meet you."

"You, too." She started toward the door, then hesitated. Even before she'd come in for the interview, she'd known she'd accept the position if it was offered to her. She needed a job, needed to support her family. If that meant traveling to the ends of the earth, she'd do it. But as she turned to walk away, Abbey realized she not only needed this position, she *wanted* it. Badly.

She loved the idea of creating her own library, building it with her own two hands. But it wasn't just the challenge of the job that excited her. She'd watched this man's eyes light up as he talked about his home. When he said Hard Luck was beautiful, he'd said it with sincerity, with passion. When he told her about the tundra and the forest, she could imagine their beauty.

"Mr. O'Halloran?" she said, surprising herself.

He was already seated, intently leafing through a sheaf of papers. He glanced up. "Yes?"

"If you decide to hire me, I promise I'll do a good job for you and the people in Hard Luck."

He nodded. "And I promise I'll phone you soon."

"WELL?" SCOTT LOOKED at Abbey expectantly when she walked into the house. "How'd the interview go?"

Abbey slipped off her pumps and curled her toes into the carpet. "Fine—I think."

"Will you get the job?"

Abbey didn't want to build up her son's hopes. "I don't know, honey. Where's Missy?" Since she paid the teenage baby-sitter top dollar, she expected her to stay with Scott and Susan for the arranged number of hours.

"Her mother wanted her to put a roast in the oven at four-thirty. Susan went with her. They'll be back soon."

Abbey collapsed into her favorite chair and dangled her arms over the sides. Her nylon-covered feet rested on the ottoman.

"Are you finished with your homework?" she asked.

"I don't have any. There's only a couple more weeks left of school."

"I know."

Abbey dreaded the summer months. Every year, day camp and baby-sitting were more and more expensive. Scott was getting old enough to resent having a teenager stay with him. Not that Abbey blamed him. Before she knew it, her son would be thirteen himself.

"Would it be all right if I went over to Jason's house?" he asked, looking eager. "I promise I'll be back in time for dinner."

Abbey nodded, but she knew it wasn't the other boy he was interested in seeing. It was those puppies that'd captured his nine-year-old heart.

SAWYER WALKED into the long, narrow mobile structure that sat next to the gravel-and-dirt runway. The mobile served as the office for Midnight Sons. Eventually they hoped to build a real office. That had been on the schedule for the past eight years—ever since they'd started the business. During those years, Charles and Sawyer had each built his own home. Sawyer's was across the street from Christian's place, which had been the O'Halloran family home. Charles's house was one street over—not that there were paved streets in Hard Luck.

But they'd been too busy running Midnight Sons—flying cargo and passengers, hiring pilots, negotiating contracts and all the other myriad responsibilities that came with a business like theirs. Constructing an office building was just another one of those things they hadn't gotten around to doing.

Exhausted, Sawyer plunked himself down on the hard-backed swivel chair at Christian's desk. Cleaning those old cabins was proving to be hard work. Much more of this, he thought ruefully, and he was going to end up with dishpan hands.

What surprised him was the willingness of their pilots to pitch in and make those old cabins livable. One thing was certain, the log structures were solid. A few minor repairs, lots of soapy water and a little attention had done wonders. Not that a forty-year-old log cabin was going to impress a city girl. More than likely, the women Christian hired would take one look at those dingy one-room shanties and book the next flight south.

The phone pealed and Sawyer reached for it. As he did, he noticed the message light blinking.

"Midnight Sons."

"Where have you been all day?" Christian grumbled. "I've left three messages. I've been sitting here waiting for you to call me back."

"Sorry," Sawyer muttered, biting back the temptation to offer to trade places. While Christian was gallivanting all over kingdom come securing airplane parts, talking to travel agents, *meeting women* and generally having a good time, Sawyer had been wielding a mop and pail. In Sawyer's opinion, his younger brother had gotten the better end of this deal. As for himself, he'd seen enough cobwebs in the past week to last him a lifetime.

"You can tell Duke I found him a blonde," Christian announced triumphantly. "Her name's Allison Reynolds, and she's going to be our secretary—well, maybe."

Sawyer's jaw tightened in an effort to hold back his irritation. "What're her qualifications?"

"You mean other than being blond?" Christian asked, then chuckled. "I'm telling you, Sawyer, I've never seen anything like this in my life. I placed the ad in the Seattle paper, and the answering service has been swamped with calls. There are a lot of lonely women in this world."

"Does our new secretary know she'll be living in a log cabin *without* the comforts of home?"

"Naturally I told her about the cabin, but, uh, I didn't have a chance to go into all the details."

"Christian! That's hardly a detail. She'll be expecting to see modern plumbing, not a path to the outhouse. Women don't like that kind of surprise."

"I didn't want to scare her off," he argued.

"She deserves the truth."

"I know, I know. Actually I offered her the position and she's thinking it over. If she does decide to accept the job, I'll give her more information."

"You mean to tell me that out of all the women who applied, you chose one who wasn't sure she wanted the job?" Sawyer was having a problem holding onto his temper. He didn't often fly off the handle, but his brother was irritating him something fierce.

"Trust me, Allison wants the position," Christian insisted. "She just needs to think about it. I would, too, in the circumstances." He paused. "Our ad was a good one. It certainly attracted a lot of attention."

Sawyer had carefully gone over the advertisement they'd submitted to the newspapers. He'd been concerned that they not inadvertently put in anything that might be misleading or violate the antidiscrimination laws. So there was nothing in the ad to suggest a man couldn't apply. No one wanted to deal with a lawsuit over this a few weeks down the road.

"I must have talked to at least thirty women in the past couple of days," Christian said, his voice ringing with enthusiasm. "And there were that many more phone inquiries."

"What about a librarian? Has anyone applied for that?"

"A few, but not nearly as many as for the position of secretary. The minute I met Allison—"

"Does she type?"

"She must," Christian answered. "She works in an office."

"Didn't you give her a typing test?" Sawyer asked, not bothering to conceal his disgust.

"What the hell for? It isn't like she'll need to type a hundred words a minute, is it? You seem to have forgotten I'm set up in a hotel. What was I going to have her type on?"

Sawyer rubbed a hand over his face. "I can't believe I'm hearing this."

"Wait until you meet her, Sawyer," Christian said happily. "She's a knockout."

"Oh great." He could picture it already. His crew would be hanging around the office, lollygagging over a dizzy blonde, instead of flying. They didn't need this kind of trouble.

"Don't get your nose bent out of joint," his brother advised. "I've made a lot of progress. You should be pleased."

"It doesn't sound like you've done much of anything." Sawyer was fuming. He'd hoped—obviously a futile hope—that Christian would use a bit of common sense.

"Listen, I haven't made up my mind about which woman to hire for our librarian. There were a couple of excellent applicants."

"Any blondes?" Sawyer asked sarcastically.

"Yeah, one, but she looked too fragile to last. I liked her, though. There's another one who seemed to really want the job. It makes me wonder why she'd leave a cushy job here in Seattle for Hard Luck. It's not like we're offering great benefits."

"But a house and twenty acres *sounds* like a hell of a lot," Sawyer said between clenched teeth.

"You think I should hire her?"

He sighed. "If she's qualified and she wants the job, then by all means, hire her."

"Great. I'll give her a call as soon as we're finished and make the arrangements."

"Just a minute." Sawyer pushed the hair off his forehead. "Is she pretty?" He was beginning to lose faith in his brother's judgment. Christian had already decided on a secretary, and he hadn't a clue if she could so much as file. Heaven help them all if he hired the rest of the applicants based on their looks, rather than their qualifications.

Christian hesitated. "I suppose you could say the librarian's pretty, but she isn't going to bowl you over the way Allison will. She's just sort of regular pretty. Brown hair and eyes, average height. Cute upturned nose.

"Now with Allison, well, there's no comparison. We're talking sexy here. Just wait until John gets a looks at her . . . front," Christian said, and chuckled. "She's swimsuit-issue material."

"Hire her!" Sawyer snapped.

"Allison? I already have, but she wants twenty-four hours to think it over. I told you that."

"I meant the *librarian*."

"Oh, all right, if you think I should."

Sawyer propped his elbows on the desk and shook his head. "Is there anything else you called to tell me about?"

"Not much. I'm not doing any more interviews for now. Allison and the librarian, plus the new teacher, that's three—enough to start with. Let's see how things work out. I've collected a couple of dozen résumés, and I'll save them for future reference."

"Don't hire any more," Sawyer insisted. He was well aware that he sounded short-tempered, but frankly he was and he didn't care if his brother knew it.

"Oh, yes, I meant to tell you. If Allison does decide to take the job, she won't be able to start right away. Apparently she's booked a vacation with a friend. I told her it's okay. We've waited this long. Another couple of weeks won't matter."

"Why don't you ask her if next year would be convenient?"

"Very funny. What's wrong with you, big brother? You sound like you're envious, not that I blame you. I wish we'd thought of this a long time ago. Meeting and talking to all these women is really great. See you."

The phone went dead in Sawyer's hand.

ABBEY'S SPIRITS were low. Dragging-in-the-gutter low. She hadn't got the job. O'Halloran would have phoned by now if he'd decided to hire her.

Scott and Susan, ever sensitive to her moods, pushed their dinner around their plates. No one seemed to have much of an appetite.

"It doesn't look like I got the job in Alaska," she told them. There wasn't any reason to keep her children's hopes alive. "Mr. O'Halloran, the man who interviewed me, would've phoned before now if he'd chosen me for the job."

"That's all right, Mom," Scott said with a brave smile. "You'll find something else."

"I wanted to move to Alaska," Susan said, her lower lip trembling. "I told everyone at school we were going to move."

"We are." Abbey knew this was of little comfort, but she threw it in, anyway. "It just so happens that we won't be moving to Alaska."

"Can we visit there someday?" Scott asked. "I liked what we read in the books you brought home. It sounded like a great place."

"Someday." *Someday,* Abbey realized, could be a magical word, filled with the promise of a brighter tomorrow. At the moment, though, the word just sounded bleak.

The phone rang, and both Susan and Scott twisted around, looking eagerly toward the kitchen wall. Neither moved. Abbey didn't allow the dinner hour to be disrupted by phone calls.

"The machine will pick up the message," she told them unnecessarily.

After the fourth ring, the answering machine automatically clicked on. Everyone went still, straining to hear who'd phoned.

"This is Christian O'Halloran."

"Mom!" Scott cried excitedly.

Abbey flew across the kitchen, ripping the phone off the hook. "Mr. O'Halloran," she said breathlessly, "hello."

"Hello," Christian responded. "I'm glad I caught you."

"I'm glad you caught me, too. Have you made your decision?" She hated to sound so eager, but she couldn't help herself.

"You've got the job, if you still want it."

"I do," Abbey said, giving Scott and Susan a thumbs-up sign. Her son and daughter stabbed triumphant fists in the air.

"When can you start?"

Abbey was certain the library would let her leave with minimal notice. "Whenever it's convenient for you."

"How about next week?" Christian asked. "I won't return from my business trip for another few weeks, but I'll arrange for my brother, Sawyer, to meet you in Fairbanks."

"Next week?"

"Will you need more time?"

"No, no," she said quickly, fearing he might change his mind otherwise. She could take the kids out of school a couple of weeks early, she wouldn't need much time to pack their belongings. Her mother would help, and what they didn't take with them on the plane she could have shipped later.

"Great. I'll see you in Hard Luck."

"Thank you. I can't tell you how pleased I am," she said. "Oh, before I hang up . . ." she began, thinking she should probably mention the fact that she'd be bringing Scott and Susan with her. Despite the provision of housing, there was nothing on the application about children.

"I'll be with you in a minute, Allison," Christian said.

"Excuse me?"

"My dinner date just arrived," he announced. "As I explained, my brother will meet you in Fairbanks. I'll have the travel agency call you to make the arrangements for your ticket."

"You're paying my airfare?"

"Of course. And don't worry about packing for the winter. You can buy what you need once you arrive."

"But—"

"I wish I had more time to answer your questions," he said distractedly. "Sawyer's really the one who can tell you what you need to know."

"Mr. O'Halloran—"

"Good luck in Hard Luck, Abbey."

"Thank you." She gave up trying. He'd learn about Scott and Susan when he returned. As far as she was concerned, the town was getting a great librarian—plus a bonus!

"YOU SURE you don't want me to fly in and meet the new librarian this afternoon?" John Henderson asked, straddling the chair across from Sawyer. His hair had been dampened and combed down, and it looked as if he was wearing a new shirt.

"Be my guest." You'd think Princess Diana was flying in from the way folks in Hard Luck were behaving. Duke had arrived at Ben's this morning clean shaven and spiffed up, smelling pungently of after-shave. Sawyer hid a grin. The next woman would follow in a few days, and he wondered how long it would take for folks to grow tired of these welcoming parties.

"You'll let John pick up the new librarian over my dead body," Duke barked. "We all know what happened the last time he flew a woman into Hard Luck."

"How many times do I have to tell you? That wasn't my fault."

"Forget it! I'll pick her up." Sawyer looked away from his squabbling pilots in disgust, and his gaze happened to catch the blackboard where Ben wrote out the daily lunch and dinner specials.

"Beef Wellington?" he asked.

"You got a problem with Beef Wellington?" Ben muttered belligerently. "I'm just trying to show our new librarian that we're a civilized bunch."

In Sawyer's opinion, this whole project didn't show a lot of promise. He'd bet his bottom dollar that none of these women would last the winter. The bad feeling he'd experienced when they first discussed the idea had returned tenfold.

"You talk to the Seattle newspaper yet?" Ben asked, setting a plate of scrambled eggs and toast in front of him.

"No." Sawyer frowned. The press was becoming a problem. It wasn't surprising that the newspapers had got hold of what was happening and wanted to do a story. They'd been hounding Sawyer for an interview all week—thanks to Christian, who'd given them his name. He was damn near ready to throttle his younger brother. And he was sorely tempted to have the phone disconnected; if it wasn't vital for business, he swore he would have done it already.

Now that the first woman was arriving, Sawyer regretted not discussing The Plan with their oldest brother. Although Charles was a full partner in the flight service, he was employed as a surveyor for Alaska Oil and was often away from Hard Luck for weeks on end. Like he was right now.

When he did return, Sawyer figured Charles would think they'd all lost their minds. Sawyer wouldn't blame him for that opinion, either.

"Well, the cabin's ready, anyway," Duke said with satisfaction.

After they'd scrubbed down the walls and floors, Sawyer and a few of the men had opened up the storeroom in the lodge and dug out the old furniture. Sawyer had expressed some doubt about sleeping on mattresses that had been tucked away in a storeroom for so many years, but Pearl and a number of other women—including several who were wives of pipeline maintenance workers—had seen to airing everything out. They'd assured him that aside from some lingering mustiness, there was nothing to worry about. Everything had been well wrapped in plastic.

As much as Sawyer hated to admit it, the cabin looked almost inviting. The black potbellied stove gleamed from repeated scrubbings. The women had sewn floral curtains for the one window and a matching tablecloth for the rough wooden table. The townspeople had stacked the shelves with groceries, and someone had even donated a cooler to keep perishables fresh for a few days. The single bed, made up with sun-dried linens and one thin blanket, did resemble something one might find in a prison, but Sawyer didn't say so. Pearl and her friends had worked hard to make the cabin as welcoming as possible.

When he'd stopped there on his way to Ben's for breakfast, he saw that someone had placed a Mason jar of freshly cut wildflowers on the table. Right beside the kerosene lantern and the can opener.

Well, this was as good as it got.

"How are you going to know it's her when she steps off the plane?" Ben asked, standing directly in front of him and watching him eat.

"I'm wearing my Midnight Sons jacket," Sawyer answered. "I'll let her figure it out."

"What's her name again?"

"Abbey Sutherland."

"I bet she's pretty."

His pilots gazed sightlessly into the distance, longing written clearly on their faces. Sawyer wouldn't have believed it if he hadn't seen it with his own eyes.

"I'm getting out of here before you three make me lose my breakfast."

"You sure you don't want me to ride along with you?" John asked hopefully.

"I'm sure. Damn sure." As it was, Sawyer was due to bring back the mail and a large order of canned goods for the grocery. He was flying the Baron, and he sincerely hoped Abbey Sutherland had packed light. He didn't have room for more than two suitcases, and he intended to store those in the nose.

Grabbing his jacket from the back of the chair, Sawyer headed out the door and across Hard Luck's main street toward the runway.

He could have flown into Fairbanks with his eyes closed, he'd made the flight so often. He landed, took care of loading up the mail and other freight, then—with a sense of dread—made his way to the terminal.

After checking the monitor to be sure the flight was coming in on schedule, Sawyer bought a cup of coffee and ventured out to the assigned gate.

He was surprised by how busy the terminal was for this time of year. Tourists, he guessed. Not that he was complaining. They brought a lot of money into the state. Not as much as the oil did, of course, but they certainly represented a healthy part of the economy.

Even the airport was geared toward impressing tourists, he noted. The first thing many saw when they walked in was a massive mounted polar bear, reared up on its hind legs. Although he'd seen the sight a hundred times, Sawyer still felt awed by it.

The plane arrived on schedule. Sipping coffee, Sawyer waited for the passengers to enter the terminal.

He glanced at each one, not knowing what to expect. Christian's description of Abbey Sutherland sure left something to be desired. From what he remembered, Christian had said she was "regular" pretty.

Every woman he saw seemed to match that description. With the exception of one.

A young woman stepped into the terminal with two kids at her side and looked around expectantly. The little girl, who couldn't have been more than six or seven, clutched a stuffed bear to her chest. The boy, perhaps two or three years older, looked as if he needed a leash to hold him back. The kid was raring to go.

The woman wasn't just pretty, Sawyer decided, she was downright lovely. Her thick brown hair was short and straight and fell to just below her ears. Her eyes skirted past him. He liked their warm brown color and he liked her calm manner.

He also liked the way she protectively drew her children close together as she looked around. She too, it seemed, was seeking someone.

With a determined effort, Sawyer pulled his gaze away from her and scanned the crowd for Christian's librarian.

Brown hair and cute upturned nose.

His gaze returned to the woman with the two children. Their eyes met, and her generous mouth formed a smile. It wasn't a shy smile, or a coy one. It was open and friendly, as if she recognized him and expected him to recognize her.

Then she walked right over to him. "Hello," she said.

"Hello." Fearing he'd miss the woman he'd come to meet, his eyes slid past hers to the people still disembarking from the plane.

"I'm Abbey Sutherland."

Sawyer's gaze shot back to her before dropping to her two children.

"These are my children, Scott and Susan," she said. "Thank you for meeting us."

CHAPTER THREE

"YOUR CHILDREN?" Sawyer repeated.

"Yes," Abbey said. It was easy to see the family resemblance between Sawyer and Christian O'Halloran. Both were tall and lean and rawboned. If he'd lived a hundred years earlier, he would've been on horseback, riding across some now-forgotten range. Instead, he was flying over a large expanse of wilderness, from one fringe of civilization to another.

Whereas Christian had been clean shaven, Sawyer had a beard. The dark hair suited his face. His eyes were a pale shade of gray-blue, not unlike those of a husky, Scott's favorite dog. He wore a red-checkered flannel shirt under a jacket marked with the Midnight Sons logo. She suspected he had no idea how attractive a man he was.

"Hi," Scott said eagerly, looking up at Sawyer.

The pilot held out his hand and she noticed that his eyes softened as he exchanged handshakes with her son. "Pleased to meet you, Scott."

"Alaska sure is big."

"That it is. Hello, Susan," Sawyer said next, holding his hand out to her daughter. The girl solemnly shook it, then glanced at Abbey and smiled, clearly delighted with this gesture of grown-up respect.

"Could we speak privately, Ms. Sutherland?" Sawyer asked. The warmth and welcome vanished from his eyes as he motioned toward the waiting area. He walked just far enough away so the children couldn't hear him. Abbey followed, keeping a close eye on Scott and Susan.

"Christian didn't mention that you have children," Sawyer said without preamble.

"He didn't ask. And there was no reference to family on the application or the agreement Christian mailed me. I did think it was a bit odd, considering that you're providing housing."

"You might have said something." An accusatory look tightened his mouth.

"I didn't get a chance," she explained in even tones. His attitude was beginning to irritate her. "I did try, but he was busy, and I really didn't think it would matter."

"There's nothing in the agreement about children."

"I'm aware of that," Abbey said, striving to keep the emotion out of her voice. "As I already told you, I filled out the application form and answered every question, and there wasn't a single one about dependants. Frankly, I don't think they're anyone's concern but mine. I was hired as a librarian. And as long as I do my job, I—"

"That's right, but—"

"I really can't see that it matters whether or not I have a family to support."

"What about your husband?"

"I'm divorced. Listen, would you mind if we discussed this another time? The children and I are exhausted. We landed in Anchorage late last night and were up early this morning to catch the connecting flight to Fairbanks. Would it be too much to ask that we wait until a more opportune moment to sort this out?"

He hesitated, then said in crisp tones, "No problem."

The pulse in his temple throbbed visibly, and Abbey suspected that it was, in fact, very much of a problem.

"I brought the Baron," he said, directing the three of them toward the luggage carousel. "All I can say is I hope you packed light."

Abbey wasn't sure how she was supposed to interpret "packed light." Everything she and the children owned that would fit was crammed into their suitcases. What hadn't gone into their luggage had been handed over to a shipping company and would arrive within the month. She hoped.

"Look, Mom," Scott said, pointing at the wall where a variety of animal trophies were displayed. Abbey shuddered, but her son's eyes remained fixed on the head of a huge brown bear. Its teeth were bared threateningly.

"That silly bear stuck his head right through the wall," Sawyer joked.

Scott laughed, but Susan stared hard as if it just might be possible.

When they'd collected all the luggage, Sawyer stepped back and gave her a disapproving glare. "You brought six suitcases."

"Yes, I know," Abbey said calmly. "We needed six suitcases."

"I don't have room for all those in the plane. I'm not exactly sure how I'm going to fit you, two kids, the mail and the rest of the cargo, much less enough luggage to sink a battleship. If you'd let me know, I could have brought a larger plane."

Abbey bit back a sarcastic reply. She'd *tried* to tell Christian about her children, but he'd been far too interested in his dinner date to listen to her. She hadn't purposely hidden anything from him or Sawyer. And, good grief, how was she supposed to know how much luggage some airplane would hold?

"Never mind," Sawyer grumbled impatiently, "I'll figure it out later. Let's get going."

Abbey would've liked something to eat, but it was clear Sawyer was anxious to be on his way. Fortunately Scott and Susan, unlike their mother, had gobbled down what the airline laughably called a meal.

They loaded everything into the back of a pickup and drove around the airport to a back road that led to a number of flight service operators.

"All that stuff belongs to Mom and Susan," Scott whispered conspiratorially as Sawyer helped him out of the cab. "They're the ones who insisted on bringing *everything*."

"Sounds just like a couple of women," Sawyer muttered. He led them to the plane.

Abbey wasn't sure what she'd expected, but this compact dual-engine aircraft wasn't it. She peeked inside and realized that what Sawyer had said was true. There was barely room for her, let alone the children and all their luggage.

"There's only three seats," she said, looking nervously at Sawyer. It didn't take a rocket scientist to figure out that three seats wasn't enough for four people.

"You'll have to sit on my desk—the seat beside mine," Sawyer instructed after climbing aboard the aircraft. "And I'll buckle the kids together on the other seat."

"Is that legal?"

"Probably not in the lower forty-eight," he told her, "but we do it here. Don't worry, they'll be fine." He moved toward the cockpit, retrieved a black binder and a stack of papers from the passenger seat and crammed them into the space between the two seats.

"Go on in and sit down," he said, "while I see to the kids."

Abbey climbed awkwardly inside and carefully edged her way forward. By the time she snapped the seat belt into place, she was breathless.

Sawyer settled Scott and Susan in the remaining seat behind her. One look at her children told Abbey neither was pleased with the arrangement. But it couldn't be helped.

"What about our luggage?" she asked when Sawyer slipped into the seat next to her.

He placed earphones over his head, then reached for the binder and made a notation in it.

"Our luggage?" she repeated.

"The suitcases don't fit. We're going to have to leave them behind."

"What?" Abbey cried. "We can't do that!"

Sawyer ignored her and continued to ready the plane for takeoff.

"How long is the flight?" Scott asked.

"About an hour."

"Can I fly the plane?"

"Not this time," Sawyer responded absently.

"*Later* can I?"

"We'll see."

"Mr. O'Halloran," Abbey said with a heavy sigh, "could we please discuss the luggage situation?"

"No. My contract is to deliver the mail. That's far more important. I'm not going to unload cargo for a bunch of silly female things you aren't going to need, anyway."

Abbey gritted her teeth. "I didn't bring silly female things. Now if you'd kindly—"

Sawyer turned around and looked at Scott. "Do you like dogs?"

Scott's eyes grew huge. "You bet I do," he answered breathlessly.

Sawyer adjusted a number of switches. "When we get to Hard Luck, I'll take you over to meet Eagle Catcher."

"Is he a husky?"

"Yup."

"Really?" Scott sounded as if he'd died and gone to heaven. He was so excited it was a wonder he didn't bounce right out of the seat.

"Um, about our luggage?" Abbey hated to be a pest, but she didn't like being ignored, either. It might be unimportant to Buck Rogers here, but she'd rather they arrive in Hard Luck with something more than the clothes on their backs.

He didn't bother to answer. Instead, he started the engines and chatted in friendly tones with a man in the control tower. Come to think of it, he chatted in friendly tones with everyone but her.

Before Abbey could protest further, they were taxiing toward the runway.

In no time they were in the air. Above the roar of the twin engines, Abbey could hear nothing except the pounding of her heart. She'd never flown in a plane this small, and she closed her eyes and held on tightly as it pitched and heaved its way into the clear blue sky.

"Wow," Scott shouted. "This is fun."

Abbey didn't share his reaction. Her stomach did a small flip-flop as the plane banked sharply to one side. She braced her hands against the seat, muttering, "Come on! Straighten up and fly right, can't you?"

Still talking to the tower, Sawyer glanced at her and grinned. "Relax," he said. "I haven't been forced to crashland in two or three months now."

"In other words, I haven't got a thing to worry about." Abbey shouted to be heard above the engines. She peeked over her shoulder to be sure Scott and Susan weren't frightened. They weren't—quite the opposite. They smiled at her, thrilled with their first small-plane ride. She, on the other hand, preferred airplanes that came equipped with flight attendants.

Abbey wasn't able to make out much of the landscape below. She'd been disappointed earlier; during the flight between Anchorage and Fairbanks Mount McKinley had been obscured by clouds. The pilot had announced that the highest mountain in North America was visible less than twenty percent of the time. He'd joked that perhaps it wasn't really there at all.

She glanced away from the window and back at Sawyer. He'd already demonstrated a fairly flexible attitude to safety rules, in her view. Now he took out the black binder he'd wedged between their seats and began to write. Abbey stared at him. Not once did his eyes shift from his task, whatever it was.

A light blinked repeatedly on the dashboard. Abbey knew nothing about small planes, but she figured if a light was blinking, there had to be a reason. They must be losing oil or gas or altitude or *something*.

When she couldn't stand it any longer, she gripped his arm and pointed to the light.

"Yes?" He looked at her blankly.

She didn't want to shout for fear of alarming her children, so she leaned her head as close to his as possible and said in a reasonable voice, "Something's wrong. There's a light flashing."

"Yes, I see." He continued writing.

"Aren't you going to do something about it?"

"In a couple of minutes."

"I'd rather you took care of it now."

"There's nothing to worry about, Ms. Sutherland—Abbey," he said. Lines crinkled around his eyes, and he seemed almost to enjoy her discomfort. "All it indicates is that I'm on automatic pilot."

She felt like a fool. Crossing her arms, she wrapped what remained of her dignity about her and stared out the window.

Sawyer tapped her on the shoulder. "You don't need to worry about your luggage, either. I've arranged with another of the flight services to have it delivered this afternoon."

He might have said something sooner, instead of leaving her to worry. "Thank you."

He nodded.

"What's that?" Scott shouted from behind her.

Abbey looked down to discover a streak of silver that stretched as far as the eye could see.

"That's the Alaska pipeline," Sawyer told Scott.

From the research she'd done on Alaska, Abbey had learned that the pipeline traversed eight hundred miles of rugged mountain ranges, rivers and harsh terrain. It ran from Prudhoe Bay to Valdez, the northernmost ice-free port in North America.

Soon Abbey noticed that the plane was descending. She studied the landscape, trying to spot Hard Luck, excited about seeing the community that would be her home. She saw a row of buildings along one unpaved street. A large structure was set off to the side. Several other buildings were scattered about. She tried to count the houses and got to twenty before the plane lined up with the runway for the final descent.

As they drew close, Abbey realized the field wasn't paved, either. They were landing on what resembled a wide gravel road. She held her breath and braced herself as the wheels touched down, sure they'd hit hard against the rough ground. To her surprise, the landing was as smooth as any she'd experienced.

Sawyer cut the engine speed and taxied toward a mobile structure near the far end of the field. Abbey strained to see what she could out of the narrow side window. She smiled when she recognized a telephone booth. In the middle of the Arctic, at the very top of the world, it was comforting to know she could call home.

A burly man who resembled a lumberjack barreled out of the mobile structure. Abbey lost sight of him, then heard the door at the side of the aircraft open.

"Howdy," he called, sticking his head and upper shoulders inside. "Welcome to Hard Luck. I'm John Henderson."

"Hello," Abbey called back.

John disappeared abruptly to be replaced by the head and shoulders of another outdoorsy-looking man. "I'm Ralph Ferris," the man announced. Three other faces crowded in around the opening.

"For the love of heaven," Sawyer snapped, "would you guys kindly let the passengers out of the plane first? This is ridiculous." He squeezed his way past her, unsnapped the seat belt secured around Scott and Susan and helped them out.

Abbey was the last person to disembark. As she moved down the three steps, she found all five men standing at attention, as if prepared for a military inspection. Their arms hung straight at their sides, their shoulders were squared, spines ramrod-straight. If any of them was surprised to see two children, it didn't show.

Muttering to himself, Sawyer stalked past Abbey and into the mobile office, leaving her alone with her children. He slammed the door as if eager to be rid of the lot of them.

Abbey felt irritation swirl over her. How could he just abandon her? How could he be so *rude?* What had she done that was so almighty terrible? Well, she could be rude, too!

"Welcome to Hard Luck." Her angry thoughts were swept aside as a tall, thin older woman with gray hair cut boyishly short stepped forward to greet her. "I'm Pearl Inman," she said, shaking Abbey's hand enthusiastically. "I can't tell you how *pleased* we are to have a librarian in Hard Luck."

"Thank you. These are my children, Scott and Susan. We're happy to be here." Abbey noted that Pearl seemed as unsurprised by the arrival of two children as the pilots were.

"You must be exhausted."

"We're fine," Abbey said politely, and indeed she felt a resurgence of energy.

"You got any kids in this town?" Scott asked, eager to make friends.

"Are there any girls my age?" Susan added.

"My heavens, yes. We had 25 students last year. I'll have one of the boys introduce you around later." She turned her attention to Susan. "How old are you?"

"Seven."

Pearl's smile deepened. "I believe Chrissie Harris is seven. Her father works for the Parks Department and serves as our PSO on the side. PSO stands for public safety officer—sort of our policeman. Chrissie will be mighty glad to have a new friend."

"What about me?" Scott asked. "I'm nine."

"Ronny Gold's about that age. You'll meet him later. He's got a bike and likes to ride all over town on it so there's no missing him."

Scott seemed appeased. "Are there any Indians around here?" he asked next.

"A few live in the area—Athabascans. You'll meet them some time," Pearl assured him.

Looking around, Abbey was surprised by the absence of snow. A large mosquito landed on her arm and she swatted it away. Susan had already received one bite and was swatting at another mosquito.

"I see you've been introduced to the Alaska state bird, the mosquito," Pearl said, then chuckled. "They're pretty thick around here in June and July. A little bug spray works wonders."

"I'll get some later," Abbey said. She'd no idea mosquitoes were a problem in Alaska.

"Come on—let's go to the restaurant and I'll introduce you to Ben and the others," Pearl said, urging them across the road toward what resembled a house with a big front porch. A huge pair of moose antlers adorned the front. "This is the Hard Luck Café. Ben Hamilton's the owner, and he's been cooking up a storm all day. I sure hope you're hungry."

Abbey grinned broadly. "I could eat a moose."

"Good," Pearl said, grinning back. "I do believe it's on the menu."

CHILDREN.

Sawyer had no one to blame but himself for not knowing that Abbey came as a package deal. He was the person who'd so carefully drawn up the application form. Apparently he'd forgotten to include one small but vital question. He'd left one little loophole. If Abbey had arrived with kids, would other women bring children, too? It was a question he didn't even want to consider.

Children.

He poured himself a mug of coffee from the office pot and took a swallow. It burned his mouth and throat, but he was too preoccupied to care. He had to figure what the hell they were going to do about Abbey Sutherland and her kids.

It wasn't that he objected to Scott and Susan. Abbey was right. Her youngsters had nothing to do with her ability to hold down the job of librarian. But the children were complications they hadn't anticipated.

First, the three of them couldn't live in the cabin. The entire space was no bigger than a large bedroom. Those cabins had never been intended as permanent living quarters. Sawyer remembered that initially he'd tried to reason with Christian and the others; no one would listen, and he'd ended up taking the path of least resistance. He'd even helped clean the cabins!

In fact, he had to admit he'd become caught up with the idea himself. It had seemed like a simple solution to a complex problem. You'd think a group of men, all of whom were over thirty, would have the brains between them to know better.

Sawyer didn't want to *think* about what his older brother would say when he found out what they'd done. Charles would be spitting nails.

Sawyer passed his hand over his eyes and sighed deeply. He didn't understand what would bring a woman like Abbey Sutherland to Hard Luck in the first place. She wouldn't last, and he knew it the moment he'd laid eyes on her.

It occurred to him that she might be running away. From her ex-husband? Perhaps she'd gotten involved in an abusive relationship. His hands formed tight fists at the thought of her husband mistreating her—at the thought of any man mistreating any woman.

Sawyer had seen for himself the dull pain in her eyes when she said she was divorced. He just wasn't sure why it was there. Understanding women wasn't his forte, and he felt himself at a real disadvantage. He lacked the experience and the expertise, but he liked to think he was a good judge of character.

Then again, maybe he wasn't. There'd been only one serious relationship in his life, and that hadn't lasted long.

Just when he was feeling comfortable with the way things were going, Loreen had started hinting marriage. Soon those hints had become ultimatums. He'd liked Loreen just fine, but he wasn't anywhere close to thinking about marriage. Once he'd told her that, she left him.

Sawyer could only assume that was the way it was with a lot of women. They wanted a ring to make everything official and complete. Well, he'd seen what could happen when a couple fell out of love. His parents were the perfect example of the kind of relationship he didn't want in his life. They'd been chained to faded dreams and unhappy memories. So Sawyer had let Loreen go, and try as he might he hadn't once regretted his decision.

Sawyer didn't know how he was going to handle the problem of Abbey and her family. What he *should* do was put her and those two kids of hers on the afternoon flight out of Hard Luck.

But he wouldn't, and he knew it. If he even suggested it, twenty men or more would take delight in lynching him from the nearest tree. Of course, they'd have to travel more than two hundred miles to find a tree tall enough for the job....

After he finished his coffee, Sawyer headed over to the café. It seemed half the town was there, eager to meet Abbey. He couldn't find a place to sit, so he stood, arms folded and one foot braced against the wall, hoping to give the impression that he was relaxed and at ease.

Ben, he noted, was pleased as a pig in ... mud to be doing such a brisk business. The beefy cook wove his way between the mismatched tables, refilling coffee cups and making animated conversation.

He lifted the glass pot toward Sawyer with a questioning look.

Sawyer shook his head. Coffee soured his stomach when he was dealing with problems.

He saw that Abbey was surrounded by four of his pilots. They circled the table where she sat with Pearl and her children, like buzzards closing in on a fresh kill. You'd think they'd never seen a woman before.

His crew was a mangy-looking bunch, Sawyer mused, with the exception of Duke, who was broad-shouldered and firm-muscled. One thing he could say about all of them was that they were damn good pilots. Lazy SOBs when the mood struck them, though. He didn't know anyone who could love flying as much as a bush pilot and still come up with some of the world's most inventive excuses to avoid duty.

Everyone plied Abbey with questions. Sawyer half expected all the attention to fluster the new arrival, but she handled their inquisition with graceful ease. It amazed him how quickly she'd picked up on names and matched them to faces.

Ben sauntered over to his side. His gaze followed Sawyer's. "Damn pretty filly, isn't she?" Ben said. "It wouldn't take much to find an excuse to marry her myself."

"You're joking." Sawyer's eyes narrowed as he studied his longtime friend.

Ben's heavy shoulders shook with silent laughter. "So that's the way it is."

"What way is that?" Sawyer challenged.

"She's already got you hooked. Before long, you'll be just like all the others, fighting for the pleasure of her company."

Sawyer snorted. "Don't be ridiculous! I just hope we don't have any more women arriving with families in tow."

Ben's eyes grew. "You didn't know about the kids?"

"Nope. Christian didn't, either, from what she said. Ms. Sutherland claims she didn't get a chance to tell him."

"Well, no one'll object to a couple more kids in Hard Luck," Ben commented.

"That's not the point."

Ben frowned. "Then what is?"

"The cabins. Abbey can't live in one of those cabins with her children."

Ben leaned against the wall with Sawyer. "Damn, but you're right. What are you going to do?"

"Hell if I know. It isn't like there's a house available for us to rent."

"Catherine Fletcher's place is vacant."

Sawyer shook his head. He wouldn't even consider approaching Catherine's family, and he doubted his brothers would be willing to do so, either, no matter what the circumstances.

The bad blood between the two families ran deep. It would take a lot more than needing an empty house to wipe out forty years of ill will.

Catherine Harmon Fletcher was in poor health now, and in a nursing home in Anchorage, close to her daughter.

Ellen, Sawyer's mother, had suffered so much unhappiness because of Catherine. But she no longer lived in Hard Luck either. She'd remarried and was living in British Columbia, as happy as Sawyer had ever known her. He didn't begrudge his mother her new life. He figured she deserved it after all the miserable years she'd endured.

"What about Pearl's? She's going to be moving in with her daughter," Ben reminded him.

Sawyer hated to see the older woman go, but she'd assured him that it was time for her to move on, especially now that her friends had mostly left.

"Pearl's not moving until we hire a replacement and she's had the opportunity to train her," Sawyer told the cook.

Ben mulled over the problem for several moments. "What about the lodge?" he asked. "I know it's been years since anyone's stayed there, but—"

"The lodge?" Sawyer repeated. "You are joking!"

"It'd take a little work."

"A little work!" Sawyer knew he was beginning to sound like a parrot, repeating everything being said, but the idea was ludicrous. The lodge was in terrible shape. It would take months of hard work and thousands of dollars to make it livable. If it hadn't been so much trouble, they would have refurbished it, instead of dealing with the cabins. Those, at least, were in one piece.

A fire had burned down part of the lodge the year their father died, and not one of the three brothers had ever had the heart to get it repaired.

Their mother had always hated the lodge, which had become a symbol of all that was wrong with her marriage, and she'd used the fire as an excuse to close it down completely. If it'd been up to him, Sawyer would've had the place torn down years ago. As it was now, the largest building in town stood vacant, a constant reminder of the father he'd loved and lost.

Ben wiped a hand across his forehead. "You're right. The lodge wouldn't work. It's a damn shame really."

Sawyer wasn't sure if Ben was talking about the abandoned lodge or Abbey's situation.

There was no easy solution. "I don't know what the hell we're going to do."

Ben was silent for quite some time, which was unusual for him. He studied Abbey and the children, then turned to Sawyer. "You could always send her back." His voice was carefully casual.

"I know."

"Are you going to?"

Sawyer felt a twinge of regret. "I can't see that we have any choice, do you?"

"It's a simple misunderstanding," Ben said. "No one's to blame. She should have told Christian about the kids."

The twinge had become an ache, and it didn't seem to want to go away. "Maybe Christian should have asked." But it didn't matter; she was here now, there was no place for her to live and *he* had to deal with it.

Better Abbey should return now, Sawyer reasoned, before he found himself making excuses for her to stay.

CHAPTER FOUR

SAWYER KNEW he wasn't going to win any popularity contests around Hard Luck if he announced that Abbey Sutherland and her children had to leave. The best way to handle the situation, he decided after giving it serious consideration, was for Abbey to back out of the deal on her own—with a little help from him.

He waited until everyone had finished eating before he worked his way over to the table where she sat with Pearl. "I'll show you to your cabin now," he offered.

She looked up at him uncertainly, as if she wasn't quite sure of his motives. "I'd appreciate that."

"Sawyer," Pearl said, placing her hand on his forearm.

Sawyer already knew what the older woman was about to say. Like him, Pearl must have realized long before now that Abbey and her children couldn't live in a dilapidated old cabin set back from town.

"When can I meet your dog?" Scott asked eagerly.

"Soon," Sawyer promised. Eagle Catcher didn't take easily to strangers; and the husky wouldn't allow the boy to come near him until after two or three visits. Sawyer decided he'd bring Scott over to the house that evening and show him Eagle Catcher's pen. But the kid would be long gone before the husky accepted him as a friend.

"I'd like to see the library, too, if it wouldn't be too much trouble," Abbey said.

"Of course," Sawyer said in a friendly voice, but a shiver of guilt passed through him. When he'd last spoken to his mother, he'd mentioned that they'd hired a librarian. Ellen had been pleased and excited to learn that her gift to the town was finally going to be put to use.

Sawyer squeezed the four of them into the cab of his pickup and drove down what was obviously the main road. There were a couple of short side streets, but none that anyone had bothered to name.

"What's that?" Susan asked, pointing to a small wooden structure that stood outside the mercantile. She giggled. "It looks like a little house on stilts."

"It's called a cache. We use it to store food and keep it safe from bears and other marauding animals."

"Alaska's got lots of bears," Scott commented as if he was well versed on the subject. "I read about them in the books Mom brought home from the library."

"How come the cache has legs that look like they're wearing silver stockings?" The question came from Susan again.

"That's tin," Sawyer explained, "and it's slippery. Discourages those who like to climb."

"I wouldn't try and climb it," Scott said.

"I don't think he's referring to young boys," Abbey told her son. "He was talking about the animals."

"Oh."

"Is it still in use?" Abbey asked.

"I understand it is. I don't know what Pete keeps in there during the summer months, but it's a crude kind of freezer in winter."

"I see."

"Oh, this is Main Street," Sawyer said as they continued down the dirt road. Dust scattered in every direction, creating a dense cloud in their wake.

"I thought there'd still be snow," Abbey said. She seemed to be trying to make polite conversation.

"It hasn't been gone all that long." Sawyer knew he should use the opportunity to tell her how harsh the winters were and how bleak life was during December, January and February, but he was afraid Abbey would see straight through him. He preferred to be a *bit* more subtle in his attempt to convince her to return to Seattle.

"Is that the school?" Scott asked, pointing to the left side of the road.

"Yup."

"It sure is small."

"Yup. We've got two teachers. One for grades one through eight and another for high school. We had more than twenty students last year."

"Ben told me you've got a new elementary teacher arriving soon," Abbey said.

"That's right." The state provided living quarters for the teacher. The house was one of the best in town, with all the modern conveniences. It was a palace compared to the cabin that would be Abbey's.

They drove past the lodge with its ugly black scars. Susan pressed her face to the window, and Sawyer anticipated another barrage of questions, but none was forthcoming.

"Is the cabin close by?" Abbey asked. They'd already passed the outskirts of Hard Luck.

"Not much farther."

She glanced over her shoulder, as if gauging the distance between the town and her new home.

Sawyer parked in front of the cluster of small cabins and pointed to the one that had been readied for her. Seeing it now, battered by time and the elements, Sawyer experienced a definite feeling of guilt. The idea of luring women north with the promise of housing and land had been a bad idea from the first.

"*These* are the cabins your brother mentioned?" Abbey kept her voice low, but her shock was all too evident.

"Yes." This was the moment Sawyer had dreaded.

"We're supposed to *live* here?" Scott asked in the same incredulous tone.

"I'm afraid so."

Susan opened the truck door and climbed out. The seven-year-old planted her hands on her hips and exhaled sharply. "It's a dump."

Sawyer said nothing. Frankly, he agreed with the kid.

"It looks like one of those places where you freeze meat in the winter, only it isn't on stilts," Scott muttered.

Without a word Abbey walked into the cabin. Sawyer didn't follow; he knew what she was going to see. A single bed, a crude table and solitary chair, along with a stove. A small store of food supplies, stacked in a primitive cupboard.

"Mom," Scott wailed, "we can't live here!"

"It is a bit smaller than what we anticipated," Abbey said. Her shoulders seemed to sink with the weight of her disappointment.

Hands still on her hips, Susan stood there, feet wide apart, as she surveyed the cabin. She shook her head. "The place is a dump," she repeated.

"Where's the bathroom?" Scott asked, giving the one-room interior a second look.

"There's an outhouse in the back," Sawyer told him. "Just follow the path."

"What's an outhouse?" Susan asked her mother.

Abbey closed her eyes briefly. "Follow Scott and you'll find out for yourself."

The two disappeared, and Abbey turned to Sawyer. He half expected her to yell at him, call him and his brother jerks for misleading her into thinking these cabins were actually livable. Instead, she asked, "What about the twenty acres?"

"It's, uh, several miles to the east of here," he explained reluctantly. "I have the plot map in the office and I'll show you later if you want."

"You mean to say the cabin doesn't sit on the twenty acres?"

"No," he answered, swallowing past his guilt. When they'd first discussed the details of this arrangement, it had all sounded equitable. Sort of. After all, Midnight Sons was picking up the women's airfare and other related expenses. But at the defeated, angry look in Abbey's eyes, Sawyer felt like a jerk. Worse than a jerk. He wished she'd just yell at him.

"I see," she said after a long silence. Her voice was so low Sawyer had to strain to hear.

He clenched his hands into tight fists to keep from taking her by the shoulders and shaking some sense into her. Was she actually thinking of staying? Christian and the others were so starved for female companionship, they'd have promised the moon to induce women to move to Hard Luck. He didn't excuse himself. He'd played a major role in this deception, too.

"I found the outhouse," Susan said, holding her nose as she returned to her mother's side. "It stinks."

"What are we gonna do?" Scott asked, sounding desperate.

"Well," Abbey said thoughtfully, "we'll just have to move a pair of bunk beds in here and add a couple of chairs."

"But, Mom..."

Sawyer glanced inside the cabin and groaned inwardly.

"We'll make it a game," Abbey told her children with forced enthusiasm. "Like pioneers."

"I don't wanna play," Susan whined.

"Maybe there's someplace else we can rent," Scott said, looking hopefully at Sawyer.

"There isn't." He hated to disappoint the boy, but he couldn't make houses that didn't exist appear out of the blue. He glanced over at Abbey, who continued to stare impassively in the direction of the cabin. He suspected she was struggling to compose herself.

"Could you show me the library now?" she finally asked. Apparently she wanted to see the whole picture before she decided. Fair enough. Sawyer hoped that once she'd had time to analyze the situation, she'd make a reasonable decision. The *only* reasonable decision.

They all piled back into the truck. On the drive out to the cabin all three Sutherlands had been filled with happy anticipation. The drive back was silent, their disappointment almost palpable.

The urge to suggest that Abbey give up and leave was almost more than Sawyer could suppress. But he'd be tipping his hand if he so much as hinted she fly home. He'd say something eventually if need be, but he'd rather she reached the conclusion herself.

The log building designated for the library had once belonged to Sawyer's grandfather. Adam O'Halloran had settled in the area in the early 1930s. He'd come seeking gold, but instead of finding his fortune, he'd founded a community.

Since the day they'd heard that Christian had hired a librarian, Sawyer and a number of other men had hauled over a hundred or more boxes of books from Ellen's house, which was now Christian's.

The original O'Halloran home consisted of three large rooms. Abbey walked inside, and once more her disappointment was evident. "I'll need bookshelves," she said stiffly. "You can't store books in boxes."

"There are several in Mother's house. I'll see that they're delivered first thing tomorrow morning."

Her gaze shot to his. "Is your mother's house vacant?"

Sawyer knew what she was thinking. "Yes and no. Mom's remarried and out of the state, but Christian lives there now. He's away at the moment, as you know."

"I see."

A young boy who introduced himself as Ronny Gold walked his bicycle up to the door and peeked inside. Scott and Ronny stared at each other.

"Can you play?" Ronny asked.

"Mom, can I go outside?"

Abbey nodded. "Don't be gone long, understand?" She glanced at her watch. "Give me a half hour or so and meet me back here."

"Okay." Both Scott and Susan disappeared with Ronny.

Hands buried deep in his pants pockets, Sawyer watched as Abbey lifted a book, studied the spine, and then reached for another. She handled each one with gentle reverence.

Sawyer waited until he couldn't bear it any longer. He'd planned to give her more time to realize she couldn't possibly live under these conditions. But if she wasn't going to admit it herself . . .

"It isn't going to work, Abbey," he said quietly. "It was a rotten idea, bringing women to Hard Luck. I blame myself. I should never have agreed to this."

"You want me to leave, don't you?" she asked in an ominously even voice, ignoring his comment.

Sawyer didn't answer her. He couldn't, because he refused to lie or mislead her any further. What surprised him most was his own realization—that he'd have liked the opportunity to know her better. Instead, he was forced to send her back to the world where she and her children belonged.

He steeled himself. Midnight Sons wasn't the only one at fault.

"You misled Christian," he said gruffly and couldn't decide who he was most angry with. Christian? Abbey? Himself?

"*I* misled Christian?" Abbey cried, her voice bordering on hysteria. "I find that insulting."

The anger that had simmered just below the surface flared to life. "You duped him into hiring you without once mentioning that you had children!" Sawyer snapped. "I realize there was nothing on the application about a family." That was one problem he was going to correct at the first opportunity. "But you should have been more honest, knowing we offered housing as part of the employment package."

"*I* should have been more honest? I find that the height of hypocrisy! I was told I'd be given living quarters and twenty acres of land, but you neglected to mention that the cabin is the size of a doghouse." She dragged in a deep breath. "How dare you suggest I broke the agreement? I'm here, aren't I?"

"You broke the spirit of our agreement."

"Oh, please! As for your free land, that's a big joke, too. You forgot to mention that it's so far from town I'd need a dogsled to reach it. If you want to talk about someone breaking the agreement, then let's discuss what you and your brother have done to me and my children."

The pain in her eyes was nearly his undoing. He had no defense, and he knew it. "All right. We made a mistake, but I'm willing to pay for your airfare home. It's the least we can do."

"I'm staying," she said flatly. "I signed a contract, and I intend to hold up my end of the bargain, despite... despite everything."

Sawyer couldn't believe his ears. "You can't."

Her eyes flashed. "Why can't I?"

"You saw the cabin yourself. There's no way the three of you could possibly live there, bunk beds or not. You might be able to manage this summer, but it'd be impossible once winter sets in."

"The children and I are staying." She said this with such determination Sawyer could readily see nothing he said or did would change her mind.

"Fine," he said brusquely. "We'll do this your way." At best, he'd give her the night. By morning she'd be sitting with her luggage at the airfield, anxious to catch the first plane out of Hard Luck. Though he doubted she'd last a full twenty-four hours.

AN HOUR LATER Abbey sat on the edge of the thin mattress and tried to think. She hadn't felt so close to breaking into tears since the day she'd filed for divorce. In some ways, the situation felt very similar to the end of her marriage. She was being forced to admit she'd made a mistake. Another in what seemed to be a very long list.

It hadn't felt like a mistake when she'd decided to accept the job. It had felt decidedly right.

The problem was that she didn't want to leave Hard Luck. She'd painted a fairy-tale picture of the town in her mind, and when it fell short of her expectations she'd floundered in disappointment. Well, she'd been disappointed before and learned from the experience. She would again.

No matter how eager Sawyer O'Halloran was to be rid of her, she was staying.

Really she had no one to blame but herself. Her father had told her the free cabin and twenty acres sounded too good to be true. She was willing to concede that he was right. But it wasn't just the promise of a home and land that had drawn her north.

She'd come seeking a slower pace of life, hoping to settle in a community of which she'd be a vital part. A community where she'd know and trust her neighbors. And, of course, the opportunity to set up and manage a library was a dream come true. She'd moved to Hard Luck because she realized her being here would make a difference. To herself, to the town, to her children most of all. She'd come so Scott and Susan would only read about drive-by shootings, gang violence and drug problems.

Although her children's reactions to the cabin had been very much like her own, Abbey was proud of how quickly the two had rebounded.

"It isn't so bad here," Scott had told her when he'd returned to the O'Halloran homestead with Ronny Gold. Susan had met Chrissy Harris, and already they'd become fast friends.

The sound of an approaching truck propelled her off the bed in a near panic. She wasn't ready for another round with Sawyer O'Halloran!

Sawyer leapt out of the cab as if he wanted to spend as little time as possible in her company. "Your luggage arrived." Two suitcases were on the ground before she reached the truck bed. Pride demanded that she get the others down herself. He didn't give her a chance.

Despite the ridiculous accusations he'd made, despite his generally disagreeable nature, Abbey liked Sawyer. She'd seen the regretful look in his eyes when he'd shown her the cabin. It might be fanciful thinking on her part, but she believed he'd wanted her to stay. He might not think it was right, or practical, or smart, but she sensed that he wanted her here. In Hard Luck.

He might pique her, irritate her, accuse her of the ridiculous, yet she found herself wishing she could know him better.

That wasn't likely, she realized. Sawyer O'Halloran had made his views plain enough. For whatever reasons, he wanted her gone.

All the suitcases were on the ground, yet Sawyer lingered. He started to leave, then turned back.

"I shouldn't have said those things earlier, about you duping Christian. It wasn't true, and I knew it."

"Is that an apology?"

He didn't hesitate. "Yes."

"Then I accept." She held out her hand.

His fingers closed firmly over hers. "You don't have to stay in Hard Luck, Abbey," he said. "No one's going to think less of you if you leave."

She held her breath until her chest started to ache. "You don't understand. I can't go back now."

Frowning, he released her hand and wiped his forearm across his brow. "Why can't you?"

"I sold my car to pay for the kids' airfare."

"I already told you I'd buy your airline tickets home."

"It's more than that."

He hopped onto the tailgate and she joined him. "I want to help you, if you'll let me."

She debated admitting how deeply committed she was to this venture, then figured she might as well, because he'd learn the truth sooner or later.

"What isn't in those suitcases is being shipped to Hard Luck. My furniture and everything I own is in the back of some truck headed for Alaska. It should arrive here within a month."

He shook his head. "It won't, you know."

"But that's what I was told!"

"Your things will be delivered to Fairbanks. There's no road to Hard Luck."

She wasn't completely stupid, no matter what he thought. "I asked Christian and he told me there was a haul road."

"The haul road is only passable in winter. It's twenty-six miles to the Dalton Highway, which doesn't even resemble the highways you know. It's little more than a dirt and gravel road. A haul road's much worse. It crosses two rivers and they need to freeze before you can drive over them."

"Oh."

"I'm sorry, Abbey, but your furniture won't go any farther than Fairbanks."

She took this latest bit of information with a resigned grimace. "Then I'll wait until winter. It's not like I have any place to put a love seat, do I?" she asked, making light of her circumstances.

"No, I guess you don't." He eased himself off the tailgate, then gave her a hand down. "I've got to get back to the field."

"Thanks for bringing our luggage by."

"Think nothing of it."

"Mom. Mom." Scott came racing toward her, his legs moving as fast as she'd ever seen them. Keeping pace with him was a large husky. "I found a dog. Look." He fell to his knees and enthusiastically wrapped his arms around the dog's neck. "I wonder who he belongs to."

"That's Eagle Catcher," Sawyer said as his eyes widened in shock. "My dog. What's he doing here? He should be locked in his pen!"

HOURS LATER, Sawyer sat in front of a gentle fire, a book propped in his hands. Eagle Catcher rested on the braided rug by the fireplace. The book didn't hold his attention. He doubted if anything could distract his mind from Abbey and her two children.

In all the years he'd lived in Hard Luck, Sawyer had only known intense fear once, and that had been the day his father died.

He never worried, but he did this June night. He worried that Susan or Scott might encounter a bear on their way to the outhouse. He worried that they'd face any number of unforeseen dangers and wouldn't know what to do.

Emily O'Halloran, an aunt he'd never known, had been lost on the tundra at the age of five. She'd been playing outside his grandparents' cabin one minute and had disappeared the next. Without a sound. Without a trace.

For years his grandmother had been distraught and inconsolable over the loss of her youngest child and only daughter. In fact, Anna O'Halloran had named the town. She'd called it Hard Luck as a result of her husband's failure to find the rich vein of gold he'd been looking for; with the tragedy of Emily's death, the name took on a new significance.

Worrying about Abbey and her children was enough to ruin Sawyer's evening. Surely by morning she'd see reason and decide to return to Seattle!

Eagle Catcher rose and walked over to Sawyer's chair. He placed his chin on his master's knee.

"You surprised me, boy," Sawyer said, scratching his dog's ears. He wouldn't have believed it if he hadn't seen it with his own eyes. Eagle Catcher and Scott had behaved as if they'd been raised together. The rapport between them had been strong and immediate. The first shock had been that the dog had escaped his pen and followed Sawyer's truck; the second, that he'd so quickly accepted the boy.

"You like Scott, don't you?"

Eagle Catcher whined as if he understood and was responding to the question.

"You don't need to explain anything to me, boy. I feel the same way." About Abbey. About her children.

He tensed. The only solution was for Abbey to leave—for more reasons than he wanted to think about. He prayed she'd use the good sense God gave her and hightail it out of Hard Luck come morning.

THE CABIN wasn't so bad, Abbey decided after her first two days. It was a lot like camping, only inside. She could almost pretend it was fun, but she longed for a real shower and a meal that wasn't limited to sandwiches.

Other than their complaints about having to use an outhouse, her children had adjusted surprisingly well.

The summer months would be tolerable, Abbey realized, but she couldn't ignore Sawyer's warning about the winter.

As for her work at the library, Abbey loved it. Sawyer had seen to the delivery of the bookcases from his mother's house, along with a solid wood desk and chair for her.

The day following her arrival, Abbey had set about categorizing the books and creating a filing system. Someday she planned to have everything up on computer, but first things first.

"How are things going?" Pearl Inman asked, letting herself into the library.

"Great, thanks."

"I brought you a cup of coffee. I was hoping to talk you into taking a short break."

Abbey stood and stretched, placing her hands at the small of her back. "I could use one." She walked to the door and looked outside, wondering about Scott and Susan, who were out exploring. It was all so different from their life in a

Seattle high rise. She knew Scott and Ronny spent a good part of each day down at the airfield pestering Sawyer.

If Scott wasn't with Ronny, then he was with Sawyer's dog. Abbey couldn't remember a time her son had been so content.

Susan and Chrissy Harris spent nearly every minute they could with each other. In two days' time they'd become virtually inseparable. Mitch Harris had stopped by to introduce himself. Mitch, Abbey remembered, worked for the Department of the Interior and was the local public safety officer. He seemed grateful that his daughter had a new friend.

"I can't believe the progress you've made," Pearl said, surveying the room. "This is grand, just grand. Ellen will be so pleased."

Abbey knew that Ellen was Sawyer's mother and the woman who'd donated the books to the town.

"I don't suppose you've seen Sawyer lately?" Pearl asked, pouring them each a cup from her thermos.

"Not a word in almost two days," Abbey admitted, hoping none of the disappointment showed in her voice.

"He's been in a bad mood from the moment you got here. I don't know what's wrong with that boy. I haven't seen him behave like this since his father died. He blamed himself, you know."

Abbey settled onto a corner of the desk and left the chair for the older woman.

"What happened to his father?"

Pearl raised the cup to her lips. "David was killed in an accident several years back. They'd flown to one of the lakes for some fishing, which David loved. On the trip home, the plane developed engine trouble and they were forced down. David was badly injured in the crash. It was just the two of them deep in the bush." She paused and sipped at her coffee.

"You can imagine how Sawyer must have felt, fighting to keep his father alive until help arrived. They were alone for two hours before anyone could reach them, but it was too late by then. David was gone."

Abbey closed her eyes as she thought of the stark terror that must have gripped Sawyer, alone in the bush with his dying father.

"If I live another sixty years I'll never forget the sight of Sawyer carrying his father from the airfield. He was covered in David's blood and refused to release him. It was far too late, of course. David was already dead. We had to pry him out of Sawyer's arms."

"It wasn't his fault," Abbey whispered. "It was an accident. There was nothing he could have done."

"There isn't a one of us who didn't tell him that. The accident changed him. It changed Hard Luck. Soon Ellen moved away and eventually remarried. Catherine Fletcher grieved something fierce. That was when her health started to fail her."

"Have I met Catherine?" Abbey asked, wondering why Pearl would mention a woman other than David's wife.

"Catherine Fletcher. No . . . no, she's in a nursing home in Anchorage now. Her daughter lives there."

Pearl must have read the question in Abbey's eyes. "Catherine and David were engaged before World War II. She loved him as a teenager and she never stopped. Not even when she was married to someone else. David broke her heart when he returned from the war with an English bride."

"Oh, dear."

"Ellen never quite fit in with the folks in Hard Luck. She seemed different from us, standoffish. I don't think she meant to be, and I don't think she realized how she looked

to others. It took me a few years myself to see that it was just
Ellen's way. She was really quite shy, felt out of place. It
didn't help any when she didn't have children right away.
She tried. God knows she wanted a family. They were married almost fifteen years before Charles was born.''

"You said Catherine got married?'' Abbey asked, her
heart aching for the jilted woman.

"Oh, yes, on the rebound, almost right after David returned from the war. She gave birth to Kate nine months
later and was divorced from Willie Fletcher within two
years.''

"She never remarried?''

"Never. I thought for a time that she and David would get
back together, but it wasn't to be. Ellen left him, you see,
and returned to England. Christian was about ten at the
time. She was gone well over a year.'' She shook her head,
then sighed. "You can understand how David's death af-
fected everyone in town. Especially Sawyer.''

"Of course.''

"What I don't get is why he's upset now. He's walking
around like a bear with a sore paw, snapping at everyone.''

Abbey gaped at her. "You think it's got something to do
with me?''

"That's my guess. But what do I know?'' Pearl asked.
"I'm only an old woman.'' She drank the rest of her coffee
and stood up to leave. "I'd best get back to the clinic before someone misses me.'' The clinic was in the community
building, close to the school and the church.

She tucked the thermos under her arm. "So, are you
staying in Hard Luck or not?'' she asked, and the question
had an edge to it, as if she wasn't sure she was going to like
the answer.

Abbey told her the truth. "I'd like to stay.''

"That doesn't answer my question.''

Abbey grinned. "I'm staying."

Pearl's lined face softened into a wide smile. "Good. I'm glad to hear it. We need you, and I have a feeling Sawyer wants you to stay, too."

Abbey gave a disbelieving laugh. "I doubt that." And if it was true once, she felt certain it no longer was.

"No, really," Pearl countered. "Unfortunately that boy doesn't have the brains of a muskrat when it comes to dealing with an attractive woman." She made her way to the door. "Give him time and a little patience, and he'll come around." With a cheerful wave, Pearl left.

Abbey returned to work and was busy unloading another box of Ellen's books. Knowing what she did now, the collection took on new meaning for her. Many of the books dated from the early to mid-fifties. Those were the childless years, when Ellen had yearned for a baby. Abbey suspected that Ellen O'Halloran had gained solace from these books, that they'd substituted for the friends she hadn't been able to make in this town so far from England.

As she set a pile of Mary Roberts Rhinehart mysteries on the desk, she heard the distinctive sound of Sawyer's truck pulling up outside.

Her heart started to race, but she continued working.

He stormed into the room and stood in the doorway, his hands on his hips. His presence filled the room until Abbey felt hedged in by the sheer strength of it. "Have you decided to stay?" he demanded.

"Yes," she answered smoothly. "I'm staying."

"You're sure?"

"Yes," she said with conviction. And she *was* sure. During her conversation with Pearl, she'd made up her mind.

"Fine. You're moving."

"Where?" Abbey had been told often enough that there wasn't any other house available.

"You can stay in Christian's house. He phoned this afternoon, and he's decided to make a vacation out of this trip. I'll let him decide what to do with you when he gets home."

CHAPTER FIVE

WHAT? Abbey's eyes flashed with annoyance—and confusion. "I'm not moving into your brother's home."

The last thing Sawyer had expected was an argument. Okay, so maybe he hadn't made the offer as graciously as he should have, but he had an excuse.

The woman was driving him nuts.

Worrying about her and those two innocent kids stuck out on the edge of town had left him nearly sleepless for two nights. It wouldn't have troubled him as much had there been neighbors close at hand. But so far, the other cabins remained empty.

"You won't be there long," he said. And he'd thought he was doing her a favor! He should have known nothing with Abbey would be easy.

She picked up another of his mother's books, handling it with reverence, then added the author and title to a list. "The kids and I are doing great where we are. Really."

"There are dangers you don't know about."

"We're fine, Sawyer."

He inhaled sharply. "Why won't you move?"

Abbey's shoulders lifted in a small, impatient sigh. "It isn't *entirely* your brother's fault that he didn't know about Scott and Susan."

"True, but you aren't entirely to blame either."

"It's very thoughtful of you to offer me the house, but no thanks." She glanced up and gave him a quick smile. For a second Sawyer swore his heart was out of control, and all because of one little smile.

"All right," he said, slowly releasing his breath, "you can move into my house, then, and I'll stay at Christian's place."

"Sawyer, you're missing the point. I don't want to put anyone out of his home."

"Christian isn't there to put out."

"I realize that, but when he does return I'll have to go back to the cabin. There isn't any other place for me and the children to move. I can't see that shuffling us around from one temporary place to another is going to help."

"But—"

"We're better off making do with what we have," she said, cutting off his argument.

"Are you always this stubborn?"

Abbey's eyes widened as if his question surprised her. "I didn't realize I was being stubborn. It doesn't make any sense to play musical houses when we have a perfectly good— When we have a home now."

"The cabins were never intended to be full-time residences," he said, knotting his hands at his sides. He shouldn't admit it, especially since his brother had begun interviewing job applicants again, promising them free housing and land. Sawyer hadn't wanted him to do it, but Christian had gotten carried away with his enthusiasm. You'd think that with the Seattle press picking up on the story, Christian would reconsider his approach. At least— thank God—the reporters had stopped calling *him*. And nothing Sawyer could say seemed to dampen his brother's enthusiasm for the project. Christian was having the time of his life.

Well, when the next women started to arrive, Sawyer decided, he'd let Christian escort them to those shacks and gleefully announce that here were their new homes. He was damned if he was going to do it.

"I don't want you to think I'm being unappreciative," Abbey said.

"You're being unappreciative," he muttered. "Christian's place has all the conveniences. Surely the kids miss television."

"They don't." She hesitated and bit her lower lip. "Though I'll admit I'd like a . . . hot shower."

Sawyer could see how tempting the offer was becoming by the way Abbey chewed on her lip.

"I'm not comfortable knowing you're out on the edge of town alone," he told her. "Because of the kids. . . People in town would be mighty upset if something happened. Pearl's been at me to find you some other place to live." He didn't want her to think there was anything *personal* in his concern. "Anyway, Christian'll be gone a month or more."

"A month," Abbey repeated thoughtfully.

"Perhaps we could compromise," he said, walking forward and supporting his hands on the sides of her desk. "You could move into Christian's house or mine, whichever you decide, until one of the other women arrives. Then, perhaps you could share the place until a more viable solution presents itself." Her hair smelled of wildflowers, and he found himself struggling to keep his mind on business.

"When's the next woman due to arrive?"

"I'm not sure. Soon."

She took a moment longer to consider, then thrust out her hand. "Thank you. I accept your offer."

Relieved, Sawyer shook her hand as briefly as possible without being rude. The softness of her skin, her scent, her combination of vulnerability and fierce determination—it was all too attractive. Too disruptive. His world, so orderly and serene before her arrival, felt as if it had been turned inside out.

One thing was sure—he didn't like it.

"I'll stop by later and pick up your luggage," he said.

Her gaze moved to meet his, and she gave him another of those heart-tripping smiles. There was something so genuine and unself-conscious about it. Their eyes held a moment longer, and every muscle in his body was telling him to lean forward and kiss her. As soon as the impulse entered his mind, he sent it flying. The last thing he wanted was to become involved with Abbey Sutherland.

"Mom—" Scott burst into the room like a warlord roaring into battle—"can I have lunch at Ronny's? His mom already said it's okay."

Sawyer leapt back so fast he damn near stumbled over Eagle Catcher, who'd ambled into the room with Scott.

"Hi, Mr. O'Halloran," the boy said in a near-squeak, then looked down at the husky. His face flushed with guilt.

Sawyer looked from the dog to the boy. "How'd Eagle Catcher get out of his pen?"

Scott lowered his head.

"Scott, did you let him out of his pen?" Abbey asked.

His nod was barely perceptible. "I went to visit him and he whined and whined, and I was going to put him back, honest I was."

Sawyer crouched down so he could speak to Scott at eye level. "I know you and Eagle Catcher are good friends, and I think that's great."

"You do?" Scott's eyes rounded with surprise.

"But it's important you ask my permission before you let him out of his yard. Otherwise, I could come home and not know where he is."

"I came to visit him, but he didn't want me to leave," Scott explained. "Every time I started to go, he'd cry. I only opened the gate so I could pet him and talk to him. I must not have latched it very good, because he followed me.''

"Next time make sure the latch is secure," Abbey told him sternly.

Scott's gaze avoided Sawyer's. "I might not have closed the gate all the way on purpose.''

Sawyer struggled to hide his amusement. "Thank you for being honest about it. Next time you want to play with my dog, all you have to do is come ask me first. That won't be difficult, will it?''

"No, sir, I can do that easy.''

"Good.''

"Eagle Catcher only likes *me*, you know," Scott announced proudly. "He wouldn't leave the pen for Susan or Ronny." He closed his mouth when he realized what he'd admitted.

So the three friends had been in his yard and attempted to lure Eagle Catcher out of the fenced-off area.

"So, can I have lunch at Ronny's?" Scott asked again, obviously eager to change the subject.

"All right, but I want you to take Eagle Catcher back to his pen. Later on you and I are going to have a nice long talk about Mr. O'Halloran's dog. Understand?''

"Okay," he said sheepishly, and before she could say another word, he dashed out the door, the husky at his heels.

Sawyer chuckled. "I can't believe the way those two hit it off. It's not like Eagle Catcher to become this attached to someone.''

"I can't understand it, either," Abbey said. "I hope this doesn't develop into a problem. He's got to understand that it's your dog, and he has to obey your rules. But Scott's always loved dogs, especially huskies, and we've never been able to have one. He was crazy about Eagle Catcher from the first time he saw him.''

"The feeling appears to be mutual. Eagle Catcher's never had anyone lavish attention on him the way Scott does. They seem destined for each other, don't they?"

Abruptly Abbey looked away.

Sawyer wondered what he'd said that had caused such a startled reaction. Did she think he was talking about the two of them? If so, Abbey Sutherland was in for one hell of a surprise.

Sawyer wasn't interested in marriage. Ever. Not even to the beautiful Abbey Sutherland. He'd learned all the lessons he needed from his own experience several years before. And from his parents, who'd tried to make marriage work, but only made each other miserable. Sawyer wanted none of that.

RARELY HAD ABBEY enjoyed a shower more. She stood under the warm spray as it pelted against her skin and savored each refreshing drop.

Exhausted from a day of playing, Scott and Susan fell asleep the minute they climbed into the two single beds in Christian O'Halloran's guest bedroom.

Abbey was sleeping in the double bed in a second spare bedroom. Although Sawyer had repeatedly told her she was welcome in his brother's home, Abbey couldn't shake the feeling she was invading Christian's privacy.

It was fine for Sawyer to offer his brother's house. But Abbey couldn't help wondering if he'd happened to mention it to Christian.

After she toweled off, she dressed in jeans and a thin sweater and walked barefoot to the kitchen where she brewed herself a cup of tea. It was difficult not to make comparisons between her stark living quarters at the cabin and the simple luxuries of Christian's home.

The kitchen was large and cheery, the white walls stenciled in a blue tulip pattern. The room's warmth and straightforward charm reminded her that Ellen O'Halloran had once lived here. Her touch was evident throughout the house.

Taking her tea with her, Abbey wandered onto the front porch and sat in the old-fashioned swing. Mosquitoes buzzed about until she remembered to light the citronella candle. The evening was beautiful beyond anything she'd imagined. Birds chirped vigorously in the background. The tundra seemed vibrant with life.

Although it was nearly ten, the sky was as bright as it had been at noon. Cupping the mug in her hands, she looked across the small patch of lawn to Sawyer's house across the street.

His home clearly lacked a woman's influence. He, too, had a yard, but there were no flower boxes decorating the window ledges, no beds blooming with hardy perennials. The porch was smaller, almost as if it had been added as an afterthought.

Drawing her knees up under her chin, Abbey gazed unseeingly at the house while she reviewed her situation. She'd taken the biggest gamble of her life by moving to Hard Luck. No one had told her she was playing against a stacked deck. But the stakes were too high for her to back down now. She wouldn't. Couldn't. Somehow, she'd find the means to stay and make a good life for herself and her children.

The front door of Sawyer's house opened, and he stepped onto the front porch. He leaned against the support beam, holding a coffee mug in his hands. For what seemed a long time they did nothing but stare at each other.

As if he'd reached some sort of decision, Sawyer set the mug aside and walked across the street. "Do you mind if I join you?" he asked.

"Not at all." Abbey hoped she didn't sound as shy as she felt. She slid over so there was plenty of room next to her on the swing.

"My mother used to sit out here in the summer," Sawyer reminisced. "There were many nights I'd get ready for bed and I'd look out and see her sitting exactly where you are, swinging as if she were eighteen again and waiting for a beau."

A sadness crept into his voice, and from what little she knew about his parents' marriage, she guessed his perception could be right. His mother might well have been waiting for the man she loved to join her—the husband she'd once, and perhaps still, loved.

He seemed to have read her thoughts. "My parents didn't have a good marriage. Don't get me wrong—they rarely raised their voices to each other. In many ways I wish they had. It might have cleared the air. Instead, they practiced indifference toward each other." He hesitated and shook his head. "I don't know why I'm telling you all that. What about your parents?"

"They're great. They've had their share of squabbles over the years and still disagree now and then. But underneath it, well, all I know is that they're deeply committed to each other." She paused, thinking about how her parents had disagreed with her move to Hard Luck. "My family gave me a firm foundation, and for that I couldn't be more grateful." She hesitated, wondering how the conversation had taken on such a personal nature. "I appreciated that foundation when my marriage floundered.

"My parents were wonderful about it. They'd never liked Dick, but they'd raised me to make my own choices and gave me the freedom to learn from my mistakes without the I-told-you-so lectures." Abbey stopped, a little flustered. She hadn't meant to discuss her marriage, especially with someone she barely knew.

"Does Scott and Susan's father have contact with them?"

"No. And he hasn't paid a penny of support since he left the army. I haven't seen him in years, and neither have the kids. In the beginning I felt a lot of anger. Not so much because of the money—that isn't nearly as important as everything else. Then I realized that it's Dick's loss. He's the one who's missing out on knowing two fabulous kids, and now I just feel sorry for him."

Sawyer reached for her hand and she gripped hold of his. Tears clouded her eyes, embarrassing her. She looked away, hoping he wouldn't notice.

"Abbey, I'm sorry. I didn't mean to pry."

"You didn't. I don't know what's wrong with me. I don't generally tear up like this."

"Maybe it's because you're a long way from home."

"Are you going to start that again—telling me I should return to Seattle?" The argument had long since grown tiresome.

He didn't answer for several moments. "No." His free hand touched her cheek and brushed a thick tendril of hair aside. Their eyes met in a rush of discovery. It seemed inevitable that he would kiss her.

It had been a long time since she'd been kissed. An even longer time since she'd wanted a man to kiss her this much. Sawyer lowered his mouth to hers and she leaned forward shyly.

Abbey wasn't sure what she'd expected, but the minute Sawyer's mouth fitted over hers, she experienced a reawakening. She felt...cherished. For so long she'd been the protector, standing alone against the world, caring for herself and her children. She hadn't had time or energy to think of herself as feminine and desirable. Sawyer made her feel both.

She opened her lips to him, and he sought her tongue with his. An onslaught of need stole her breath. She felt as though she'd taken a free-fall from twenty thousand feet.

Sawyer eased his mouth from hers, then hurried back as if he needed a second kiss to confirm what had happened the first time. His gentleness produced an overwhelming ache deep inside her. One that was emotional, as well as physical. Those feelings had been so long repressed she had trouble identifying them.

Sawyer lifted his mouth from Abbey's. Slowly she opened her eyes and found him studying her. His eyes were intense with questions.

She smiled, and the simple movement of her lips appeared to be his undoing. He groaned and leaned forward, kissing her with a passion that left her breathless and weak.

Whatever happened to her in Hard Luck, whatever became of the housing situation, whatever happened between her and Sawyer from this point onward, Abbey knew that in these moments, they'd shared something wonderful. Something special.

He ended the kiss with reluctance. Abbey hid her face in his shoulder and took one deep breath after another.

They didn't speak. She sensed that words would have destroyed the magic. He gently rubbed her back.

'I'd better get back,'' he whispered after a time.

She nodded. He loosened his hold, then released her. Abbey watched as he stood, buried his hands in his pockets... and hesitated.

He seemed to want to say something, but if that was the case, he changed his mind. A moment later, he whispered a good-night and walked across the street to his own home.

Abbey had the distinct feeling that they wouldn't discuss this evening. The next time they met it would be as if nothing had happened between them.

But it had, and Abbey knew it.

AFTER AN HOUR of restlessly pacing the floor, Sawyer sat down at his desk and leafed through his personal telephone directory. He needed to talk to Christian, the sooner the better.

He ran his finger down a number of hotel listings. He didn't have Christian's itinerary, so he couldn't be sure which Seattle hotel his brother was staying at—or even if he was still *in* Seattle—but he swore he'd find him if it took the rest of the night.

He punched out a series of numbers and waited for the hotel operator to answer. As luck would have it, Christian was registered at the Emerald City Empress. The operator connected him with his brother's room.

Christian answered on the fourth ring, sounding groggy.

"It's Sawyer."

"What the hell time is it?"

"Eleven."

"No, it isn't." Sawyer could visualize his brother picking up the travel alarm clock and staring at its face. "It might be eleven in Hard Luck, but it's midnight here. What the hell could be so important that it can't wait until morning?"

"You haven't called me in several days."

"You got my message, didn't you?"

Sawyer frowned. That was what had prompted him to move Abbey into Christian's home. "Yeah, I got it. So you're going to take some personal time."

"Yeah. Mix business with pleasure. I might as well, don't you think?

"You might think of phoning more often."

Christian groaned. "You mean to say you woke me out of a sound sleep because we haven't talked recently? You sound like a wife checking up on her husband!"

"We've got problems," Sawyer insisted, gritting his teeth.

"What kind of problems?"

"Abbey Sutherland arrived."

"What's the matter? Don't you like her?"

Sawyer almost wished that was true. Instead, he liked her so damn much he'd completely lost the ability to sleep through an entire night. Either he was pacing the floor, worried about her living in that cabin alone with her two children, or he was fighting every instinct he possessed to walk across the street and make love to her. Either way, he was fast becoming a lunatic.

"I like her just fine. That's not the problem."

"Well, what is?"

"Abbey didn't arrive alone." A short silence followed his announcement. "She brought her two children."

"Now, just a minute," Christian said hurriedly. If he wasn't awake earlier, he was now. "She didn't say a word about having children."

"Did you ask?"

"No...but that shouldn't have mattered. She might have said something herself, don't you think?"

"All I know is you'd better revise the application, and damn quick."

"I'll see to it first thing in the morning." His promise was followed by the sound of a breath slowly being released. "Where's she staying? You didn't stick her in one of the cabins, did you? There's barely room enough for one, let alone three."

"She insisted that was exactly where she'd stay until I convinced her to move into your house."

"My house!" Christian exploded. "Thanks a lot."

"Can you think of anyplace else she could live?"

There was a moment's silence. "No."

"I tried to talk her into moving back to Seattle, but she's stubborn." And beautiful. And generous. And so much more.

"What are we going to do with her once I return?" Christian asked.

"I haven't got a clue."

"You're the one who told me to hire her," his brother argued.

"I did?"

"Sure, don't you remember? I was telling you about Allison Reynolds and happened to mention there were two women I was considering for the position of librarian. You said I should hire the one who wanted the job."

So apparently Sawyer was responsible for his own misery.

"Maybe she'll fall in love with John or Ralph," Christian said hopefully, as if this would solve everything. "If she gets married, she won't be our problem. Whoever's fool enough to take her on *and* her children will be responsible for her."

Anger slammed through Sawyer. He had to struggle to keep from saying something he'd later regret.

"Any man who married Abbey Sutherland would be damn lucky to have her," he said fiercely.

"Aha!" Christian's laugh was triumphant. "So that's the way it is!"

"Just how much longer do you plan to be away?" Sawyer demanded, ignoring his brother's comment. A comment that was doubly irritating because it echoed one made by Ben the very day of Abbey's arrival.

"I don't know," Christian muttered. "I've been busy interviewing more women, and I'd like to hire a couple more. I haven't even gotten around to ordering the supplies and plane parts. While I'm here, I thought I might as well take a side trip up to see Mom. She'd be disappointed if I didn't."

"Fine, go see Mom."

"By the way, Allison Reynolds decided she wanted the position, after all. Take my advice, big brother, and don't get all excited over this librarian until you meet our new secretary," Christian said. "One look at her'll knock your socks off."

"What about a health-care specialist?"

"I've talked to a number of nurses, but nothing yet. Give me time."

"Time!" Sawyer snapped. "It isn't supposed to take this long."

"What's your hurry?" Christian asked, and then chuckled. An evil sound, Sawyer thought sourly. "The longer I'm gone, the closer your librarian friend will be." Laughter echoed on the line. "Lord, I love it. You were against the idea from the beginning—and now look at you."

"I'm still against it."

"But not nearly as much as you were before you met Abbey Sutherland. Aren't I right, big brother?"

ABBEY STOOD in front of the lone store in town, popularly known as the mercantile. It was decorated in a style she was coming to think of as Alaskan Bush—a pair of moose antlers adorned the doorway. She walked inside with a list of things she needed. The supplies she'd been given when she arrived were gone. She also craved some fresh produce, but didn't know what to expect to pay for it.

A bell dinged over the door, announcing her arrival.

The mercantile was smaller than the food mart where she bought gas back in Seattle. The entire grocery consisted of three narrow aisles and a couple of upright freezers with price lists posted on the door. A glass counter in front of the antique cash register sold candy and both Inupiat and Athabascan craft items.

A middle-aged man with a gray beard and long hair tied back in a small ponytail stepped out from behind the curtain. He smiled happily when he saw her. "Abbey Sutherland, right?"

"Right. Have we met?"

"Only in passing." He held out his hand for her to shake. "I'm Pete Livengood. I own the store and have a little tourist business on the side."

"Pleased to meet you," she said, smiling back, wondering how much tourist trade he got in Hard Luck. "I've got a few things I want to pick up for dinner this evening."

"Great. Let me have a look at your list and I'll see what I can do."

Abbey watched as he scanned the sheet of paper. "We don't sell fresh vegetables here since most folks have their own summer gardens. Every now and again I'll have Sawyer bring me something back from Fairbanks, but it's rare. Wintertime's a different story, though."

"I see." Abbey had hoped to serve taco salad that evening. She knew the kids would be disappointed.

"Louise Gold's got plenty of lettuce in her garden. She was bragging to me about it just the other day. I suspect she'd be delighted if you'd take some of it off her hands."

"I couldn't ask her." Abbey had only met Ronny's mother briefly. The Gold family had been wonderful, and she didn't want to impose on their generosity any more than she had already.

"Things are different in the Arctic," Pete explained. "Folks help one another. If Louise knew you needed lettuce for your dinner and she had more than she wanted, why she'd be insulted if you didn't ask. Most folks order their food supplies a year at a time. I'll give you an order form and you can read it over. Louise can probably help you better than I can, since you're buying for a family of three."

"A *year* at a time?"

"It's far more economical that way."

"Oh."

"Don't worry about this list here. I know how hard you're working setting up the library. I'll take care of everything you have here myself, including talking to Louise about that lettuce."

"Oh, but... I couldn't ask you to do that."

"Of course you could. I'm just being neighborly. Tell you what. I'll gather everything together and deliver it myself. How does that sound?"

"Wonderful. Thank you."

"It's my pleasure," Pete said, grinning broadly as if she'd done something special by allowing him to bring her groceries.

As the day progressed, Abbey was disappointed not to see Sawyer. She found herself waiting for him, hoping he'd stop by, wondering if he'd mention the kisses they'd shared. Knowing he wouldn't.

Her kids were in and out of the library all morning. Abbey enjoyed being accessible to her children; the experience of having them close at hand for the summer was a new one.

When Abbey had first asked Pearl about day care, the older woman had thought she was joking. There was no such thing in Hard Luck. Not technically. Abbey knew that Louise Gold watched Chrissie Harris for Mitch, but there wasn't any official summer program for school-age children.

Scott and Susan throve on the sense of adventure and freedom. Their happiness seemed to bubble over.

"Hi, Mom," Scott said, strolling into the library. Eagle Catcher traipsed beside him.

"Once the library opens, we can't have Sawyer's dog inside," she told him.

"We can't?" Scott was offended on the husky's behalf. "That doesn't sound fair. I let him go everyplace else I go."

"Dogs can't read," she reasoned.

"I bet I could teach him."

"Scott!"

"All right, all right."

"Did you ask Sawyer about letting him out of his pen?"

"Yup. I went down to the airfield and he seemed real busy, and I thought he might get mad at me, but he didn't. He said I'd been patient and he was proud of me." Scott beamed as he reported the compliment. "He's short-handed 'cause his brother's gone, and he had to take a flight this morning himself. I don't think he wanted to go, but he did."

"Oh." Her disappointment was keen. "Did he say when he'd be back?"

"Nope, but I invited him to dinner. That was okay, wasn't it?"

"Ah..."

"You said we were having taco salad, didn't you?"

"Yes ... What did Sawyer say?"

"He said he'd like it just fine, but he wanted to make sure you knew about him coming. I told him you always fix lots, and I did promise to tell you. It's all right, isn't it?"

Abbey nodded. "I suppose."

"I'll go see if Sawyer's back yet. I'll tell him you said he could come." Scott raced out the door at breakneck speed,

Eagle Catcher in hot pursuit. Abbey couldn't help grinning—it took the energy of a sled dog to keep pace with her son.

She was barely aware of the afternoon slipping past until Pete Livengood stopped by with her groceries and surprised her with a small bouquet of wildflowers. His thoughtfulness touched her.

Abbey was putting everything away for the day when a shadow fell across her desk. She looked up to find Sawyer standing in the doorway, blocking the light.

He looked tired and disgruntled. "Isn't it about time you went home?"

"I was just getting ready to leave."

"Scott invited me to dinner."

"So I heard." She found herself staring at him, then felt embarrassed and looked away. Her thoughts were in a muddle as she scrambled for something to say to ease the sudden tension between them.

"Pete Livengood brought me wildflowers," she blurted, convinced she sounded closer to Susan's age than her own.

"Pete was here?"

"Yes, he delivered a few groceries. He's really a very nice man."

Sawyer was oddly silent, and Abbey tried to fill the awkward gap.

"When he stopped by, we talked for a bit. He's led an interesting life, hasn't he?"

"I suppose."

Abbey felt Sawyer stiffen at her side. "Do you have any idea how old Pete Livengood is?" he demanded.

"No." Nor did she care. In fact, she couldn't think of a reason it should matter. He was a rough-and-ready sort who'd lived in Alaska for close to twenty years. Abbey found his stories interesting and had asked a number of questions. Perhaps Sawyer objected to her spending so much time away from her job.

"Pete's old enough to be your father!"

"Yes," she said curiously. "Is that significant?"

Sawyer didn't respond. "I gave specific instructions that you weren't to be bothered."

"Pete didn't bother me."

"Well, he bothers me," Sawyer said abruptly.

"Why?"

Sawyer expelled his breath and glanced toward the ceiling. "Because I'm a bloody fool, that's why."

CHAPTER SIX

THE ATMOSPHERE in the Hard Luck Café was decidedly cool when Sawyer stopped by for breakfast.

"Morning," he greeted Ben, then claimed a seat at the counter. Three of his pilots were there, as well, and he nodded in their direction. They ignored him.

Ben poured him a cup of coffee.

"I'll take a couple of eggs, along with a stack of hotcakes." Sawyer ordered without looking at the menu tucked behind the sugar bowl.

John Henderson grumbled something Sawyer couldn't hear, slapped some money down on the counter and walked out. Ralph, who sat two stools down from Sawyer, followed suit. Duke muttered something, then he was gone, too.

Sawyer looked up, surprised. Three of his best pilots acted like they couldn't get away from him fast enough. "What? Do I have bad breath?"

Ben chuckled. "Maybe, but that ain't it."

"What'd I do?"

Ben braced his hands on the counter. "I'd say it has something to do with Abbey Sutherland."

Sawyer tensed. "What about Abbey?"

"What I hear, you had a word with Pete Livengood about him dropping off Abbey's groceries at the library."

"So what?" To Sawyer's way of thinking, the old coot had no business interrupting her when she was at work. The library wasn't open yet. Besides, Pete hadn't brought by that bouquet of wildflowers because he was interested in finding a good book to read. No, he was after Abbey. That infuriated Sawyer every time he thought about it.

Pete wasn't right for Abbey, and Sawyer wasn't planning to let him pester her while she was on his property. All right, so maybe his family *had* donated his grandfather's cabin to the town. It didn't matter; Sawyer felt responsible for her. If it wasn't for Midnight Sons, she wouldn't even be in town.

"Just remember I'm a disinterested observer," Ben said. "But I've got eyes and ears, and I hear what the men are saying."

"Okay, so what's the problem?"

Ben delivered the eggs and cakes hot off the griddle, and topped up Sawyer's coffee mug. "Ralph and John and a couple of the others object to your keeping Abbey to yourself."

Sawyer didn't see it that way. "What gives them the idea I'm doing that?"

"Wasn't it you who warned everyone to stay away from the library?"

"That isn't because I'm keeping Abbey to myself," he argued. "The woman's got work to do, and I don't want her constantly interrupted. It isn't books that interest John and the others, and you and I both know it."

"Perhaps not, but I don't remember you taking such a keen interest in your mother's collection before now."

Sawyer wasn't going to argue further, although the discussion irked him. No one seemed to appreciate what he was trying to do. "The library should be open soon, and then the men can visit as often as they like."

That seemed to appease Ben and Sawyer suspected it would appease the other men, as well.

"Next on the list of complaints," Ben continued, "the guys think you're inventing flights to keep the crew busy so you can court Abbey without interference."

"I'm not courting her," he said heatedly.

"Word is, you had dinner at her house."

"That's true, but Scott was the one who invited me." He hated having to defend his actions, but the truth was, it was the best dinner he'd had all summer. And he didn't just mean the food.

"Are you saying you don't have any personal interest in her yourself?"

"That's right." Although he didn't hesitate, Sawyer wondered how honest he was being. It was a good thing no one knew he'd been kissing Abbey.

Ben narrowed his eyes. "You're not interested in her," he repeated. "Is that why you nearly bit Pete's head off?"

Sawyer sighed, his appetite gone. "Who told you that? I didn't so much as raise my voice."

"But you made it clear you didn't want him seeing Abbey."

"Not before the library's open," Sawyer insisted. "This is the very reason I objected to the idea of recruiting women to Hard Luck in the first place. Look at us!"

"What?" Ben asked.

"A few weeks ago we were all friends. Don't you see what's happening? We're at each other's throats."

"Well, we got one thing settled, though, didn't we? You're not interested in her yourself."

"Of course not," Sawyer said stiffly.

"Then you won't mind if a few of the other guys develop intellectual interests that require research trips to the library?"

Sawyer shrugged. "Why should I care?"

"That's what I'd like to know," Ben said, and Sawyer had the feeling the old stew-burner was seeing straight through him.

"All I ask is that the guys give Abbey a little breathing room. The least they can do is wait until the library's ready."

"And when will that be?"

"Soon," he promised. "I understand she'll be ready to open it up to the public in a few days."

"Good. I'll pass the word along," Ben said, then returned to the kitchen.

Sawyer ate his breakfast, and although Ben was an excellent cook, the food rested in his stomach like a lead weight.

It didn't take him long to acknowledge that he was guilty of everything Ben had suggested. He'd gone out of his way to keep the men as far from Abbey as he could arrange. It hadn't been a conscious decision, at least not in the beginning. But it was now.

ABBEY WAS PUTTING AWAY the last of the dinner dishes the following night when she heard Scott and Susan talking on the front porch with a third person. The weather had been decidedly warm, and she'd changed into shorts when she arrived home from work. Who'd have believed it would reach the mid-eighties in the Arctic? Not Abbey.

Drying her hands on a kitchen towel, she walked onto the porch to discover Sawyer chatting with her children. Eagle Catcher stood at his side.

"Hello," he said when she joined them.

"Good evening." She'd been hoping she'd see Sawyer again soon. His eyes said he was eager for her company, too.

Being with him felt right. She loved the easy way he spoke to her children, his patience with Scott over the dog, his gentleness when it came to dealing with Susan. Her daughter had adored him from the moment he'd held out his hand to her when they'd met at the airport.

"When are we going to see the northern lights?" Scott asked Sawyer. He'd talked of little else over dinner that night. "Ronny told me it's better than the Fourth of July fireworks, but no matter how late I try to stay awake, it won't get dark."

"That's because it's early summer, Scott, and the solstice isn't even due for another two weeks. Wait until the end of August—you'll probably begin to see them then."

"Does it ever get dark in Alaska?" Susan asked.

"Yes, but for an amazingly short time in the summer. Winter, however, is another story."

"Ronny told me it's dark almost all day," Scott put in, "but I knew that from the books Mom read when she applied for the job."

"Tell me what the northern lights look like," Susan pleaded.

Sawyer sat on the swing and Susan sat beside him; Scott hunkered down next to Eagle Catcher. "Sometimes the light fills the sky from horizon to horizon. It's usually milky green in color and the colors dance and flicker. Some folks claim they can hear them."

"Can you?"

Sawyer nodded. "Yup."

"What's it sound like?"

Sawyer's eyes caught Abbey's. "Like tinkling bells. I suspect you'll hear them yourself."

"Are they always green?"

"No, there's a rare red aurora that's the most magnificent of all."

"Wow, I bet that's pretty!"

"You know, the Inuit have a legend about the aurora borealis. They believe the lights are flaming torches carried by departed souls who guide travelers to the afterlife."

Abbey sat on the edge of the swing. Soon Susan was in her lap, and she was next to Sawyer. He looked over at her and winked.

Her children seemed to have a hundred questions for Sawyer. He told them the story of how his grandfather had come to Hard Luck, following a dream, searching for gold.

"Did he find gold?" Scott asked.

"In a manner of speaking, but not the gold he'd anticipated. It was here, but he never really struck it rich. He died believing he'd failed his wife and family, but he hadn't."

"Why did he stay?" Abbey asked.

"My grandmother refused to go. They had a little girl named Emily who disappeared on the tundra, and afterward my grandmother refused to leave Hard Luck."

"Did she think there was some chance Emily would come back?"

"She never stopped looking."

"What do you think happened to her?" Scott asked.

"We can only guess, but none of the prospects are pleasant. That's why it's so important for you never to wander off on your own. Understand?"

The two children nodded solemnly.

Abbey glanced at her watch, amazed at how late it was. When she'd read that Alaska was the land of the midnight sun, she'd assumed the light would be more like dusk. She was wrong. The sun was so bright she had to prop a board against the curtains in the children's bedroom to make it dark enough for them to fall asleep. As it was, their routines had started to shift. They stayed awake later and slept in longer.

"Bedtime," she told them.

Her announcement was followed by the usual chorus of moans and complaints.

"Come on, Susan," Sawyer said, standing. "I'll give you a piggyback ride." He reached for the child and hoisted her onto his back. Susan giggled, circling her arms around his neck.

"You're next, partner," he told Scott.

"I'm too old for that stuff," Scott protested, but Abbey knew it was for show. He was as keen as his sister to have Sawyer give him a ride.

"Too old? You've got to be kidding," Sawyer said, his voice rising in exaggerated disbelief. "You're never too old for fun." Then, before Scott could escape, Sawyer gripped him around the waist and tucked him against his side.

Scott was giggling and kicking wildly. With a smile, Abbey held open the screen door, and Sawyer carried them down the hallway to the bedroom they grudgingly shared.

"How about a cup of coffee?" she asked while the children changed into their pajamas.

His eyes brightened momentarily, then he frowned and shook his head. "I can't. Thanks, anyway. I stopped over to tell you I talked to my brother about the housing situation."

Susan burst out of the bedroom wearing her Minnie Mouse pajamas and raced into the kitchen. Scott was close behind, his pajama top half over his head. When her two youngsters were this excited, it was always awhile before they settled down enough to fall asleep.

"Will you tuck me in?" Susan asked, gazing up at Sawyer.

He glanced at Abbey. "I suppose so, if your mother doesn't object."

They hopped up and down as if it were Christmas morning and they'd woken to find the tree surrounded by gifts.

Taking him by the hand, Susan led Sawyer into the bedroom. Abbey followed, her arm around Scott's shoulders. Sawyer tucked each child into bed, but it was soon apparent that neither one intended to go to sleep.

"Tell us a story," Susan pleaded, wriggling out from under the covers. She hugged her favorite doll against her.

Scott, too, seemed to think this was a brilliant idea. "Yeah," he said eagerly. "One with a dog in it." It went without saying that he would have welcomed Eagle Catcher in his bedroom had Abbey and Sawyer allowed it.

"All right, all right," Sawyer agreed. "But then you have to promise to close your eyes and go to sleep."

Sawyer entertained them with a story for the next fifteen minutes. He was obviously inventing as he went along, and Abbey was both charmed by his spontaneity and moved by his willingness to do this for her children. Afterward, emotion tugged at her heart as Sawyer bowed his head while each child recited a prayer.

A few minutes later, he slipped out of the bedroom. Abbey was waiting for him in the kitchen. She heated water in the microwave for a cup of tea.

"Thank you," she whispered, not looking at him.

There was an uncomfortable silence, then Sawyer cleared his throat. "As I said, I spoke with Christian about the housing situation. It's apparent to both of us that you and the children can't go back to the cabin."

"But I don't really have any choice, do I?"

"There's one vacant house in town." His mouth thinned. "It belonged to Catherine Fletcher."

The name was vaguely familiar, and Abbey tried to recall where she'd heard it. Then she remembered the day Pearl Inman had stopped by the library and told her about Sawyer and his family, and some of Hard Luck's background.

If she recalled correctly, the two families had been at odds since right after World War II.

"Christian suggested we contact Catherine's family. She's in a nursing home now, and it's unlikely she'll ever return to Hard Luck."

"I'd be happy to pay whatever rent she feels is fair."

"Midnight Sons will pick up the rent," Sawyer insisted. "We promised you free housing when you agreed to move here, and that's what you're going to get."

"Do you think she'll let me have the house?" Abbey asked hopefully.

Sawyer frowned. "She's a cantankerous old woman, and it'd be just like her to refuse out of pure spite. I'm hoping I don't have to speak to her at all. Her daughter's far more reasonable."

"You don't like Catherine?"

"No," Sawyer said without emotion. "She went out of her way to hurt my mother, and I don't find that easy to forgive. It's a long story better left untold."

Despite his negative feelings toward the old woman, Sawyer was willing to approach her on Abbey's and the children's behalf. Every day Abbey found a new reason to be grateful for Sawyer's presence in her life.

"I appreciate what you're doing," she murmured. "Are you sure you don't have time for coffee?"

His eyes held hers, and a warm, unfamiliar sensation skittered through her. Hastily he shook his head. "I've got to get back." He looked past her down the hallway that led to the bedrooms. "You were right when you said your husband was the one to be pitied. Scott and Susan are great kids. They'd make any man proud."

He moved past her, then paused on his way out the door and kissed her. Only their lips touched. The kiss was brief and casual, as if they exchanged such an intimacy every day.

It didn't strike Abbey as unusual until he'd left the house. She pressed her fingertips to her lips and watched him from the screen door.

His steps seemed to have an uncharacteristic bounce as he walked down the stairs. He was halfway across the narrow dirt road when he appeared to realize what he'd done. He stopped abruptly and whirled around.

"Good night, Sawyer," she called.

He raised his hand in farewell, then continued across the street to his own home.

"MIDNIGHT SONS," Sawyer barked into the telephone receiver, stretching the cord as far as it would go so he could reach a pad of paper.

"Sawyer, it's Christian. Listen up. Allison Reynolds is on her way."

Sawyer blinked. "Who?"

"Our new secretary. I talked to her this morning, and she's back from her vacation and ready to start work first thing Monday morning."

"Great. This is the woman who doesn't type, right?"

"She won't need to. Besides, there's more to being a secretary than typing. Don't worry, what she lacks in one area she makes up for in others."

"Have you booked her flight?"

"Yeah. She's coming in on Friday morning. Same flight Abbey Sutherland did."

Sawyer wrote down the information. "I'll send Duke in to meet her," he said. That should help quell some of the dissension among the men.

"Not Duke," Christian protested. "Send Ralph."

"Why not Duke?"

"He'll talk her head off, and you know what a chauvinist he can be. I don't want Allison's first impression of Hard Luck to be negative."

"All right, all right, I'll send Ralph."

"Ralph," Christian repeated the pilot's name slowly. "Maybe John would be better," he suggested.

John? It was his big mouth that scared off the last teacher! "Why not Ralph?"

"He's too eager, you know? He might say something that would offend Allison."

"Why don't you get your butt home so you can pick her up yourself?" It seemed to Sawyer that his brother was being *much* too particular.

"I would if I could get there in time. I've interviewed a nurse I think would be excellent. I know you asked me to wait on hiring anyone else, but this gal is perfect."

"Do it." If she met the qualifications, Sawyer couldn't understand the problem.

"She's older. Way older. Pete Livengood's age."

"So?" All the better as far as Sawyer was concerned. Then maybe Pete would stop showing an interest in Abbey.

"I was hoping to find someone younger. Attracting women to Alaska isn't as easy as it sounds. I get lots of calls, but once they hear exactly how *far* north we are, they start asking a lot of questions." He paused. "I had to do some fast talking to convince Allison to give us a try."

"Every position can't be filled with Allison Reynolds clones," Sawyer said testily.

"I know. I know. Listen, I'll talk to you again soon as I can. I'll want to know how Allison is adjusting."

"Fine."

"Any word from Charles lately?"

"None, but I expect he'll show any day, hungrier than a bear and meaner than a wolverine." Their eldest brother kept his own hours. He was often gone for weeks at a time, then would blow into town with his geological equipment and stay for a month or two. There was a restlessness in Charles that never seemed to ease. Sawyer didn't question it, but he didn't understand it, either.

He spoke to his younger brother for only a few more minutes. Sawyer hung up the phone to find John Henderson standing on the other side of the desk.

"You got a minute?" the pilot asked nervously.

Sawyer nodded. "Sure. What's the problem?"

"Not a problem as such. It's more of a . . . concern."

"Sit down." Sawyer motioned toward the vacant chair.

"If you don't mind, I prefer to stand," the other man said stiffly.

Sawyer arched his eyebrows and leaned back in his chair. "Suit yourself."

John folded his hands. He seemed to need a couple of minutes to gather his thoughts. Finally he blurted, "Me and a few of the other guys aren't happy with the way things are going around here."

"What things?"

Once more it appeared that John was having difficulty speaking his mind. "You've got an unfair advantage, and it's causing hard feelings."

Now Sawyer understood. After his talk with Ben, he should've realized sooner that this discussion wasn't about Midnight Sons at all. John had come to talk to him about Abbey.

"You're upset because I asked you not to disturb the new librarian while she organizes the library."

"Yes," he said angrily. "You ordered us to stay away until the library's open, but I notice the same doesn't apply to you."

"I'm her contact person," Sawyer explained evenly. "She needs someone who can help her, answer questions and so on."

"Let me be her contact person," John argued. "Or Duke. None of us would pester her. We just want to drop by the library and make her feel welcome. That sort of thing. Everyone knows what happened when Pete made the mistake of visiting her. It wasn't right that you should chew him out for doing his job."

"Pete delivers groceries now? That's news to me."

"Come on, Sawyer, get real. If Abbey stopped by here and needed something, wouldn't you be willing to take it to her?"

Before Sawyer could respond, John continued.

"Of course you would. She's pretty and she's nice, and hell, I thought when we came up with the idea of bringing women to Hard Luck, we'd at least get to talk to them now and then."

Sawyer released a lengthy sigh. "Perhaps I have been a bit overprotective."

John's jaw tightened. "The guys are saying you want her for yourself."

Sawyer opened his mouth to disagree, then realized they had more than enough evidence to hang him. "You could have a point there."

"That's what we think. All we're asking is that you drop the restrictions on the rest of us. It's only fair, don't you think? You have my word of honor that I won't pester her, and I don't think the others will, either."

Sawyer couldn't see any choice. If he didn't do it, he was likely to have a mutiny on his hands. "All right," he said reluctantly.

John relaxed. "No hard feelings?"

"None," Sawyer assured him. He reached for his pad of paper and peeled off the flight information Christian had given him. "In fact, we've got another woman due to land on Friday. Would you be willing to pick her up?"

"Would I?" John's face broke into a wide grin not unlike the expression on Scott's face when Sawyer had given him permission to play with Eagle Catcher.

The pilot quickly composed himself. "I'll have to check my schedule."

"Great. Do that and get back to me."

ABBEY HAD NO IDEA what was happening. She'd had four visitors in the past hour. Each had produced a valid reason for coming to the library. She hadn't realized how eagerly awaited the opening of the library was. In light of such overwhelming interest, she decided to do just that the next morning.

Abbey finished for the day and collected her things. She'd been visited by everyone but the one person she was aching to see. Sawyer.

As she walked toward Christian's house, she recognized the familiar sound of his pickup behind her. She turned and waved.

He slowed to a crawl. "Heading home?"

"Yeah."

"How about a ride?"

She laughed. "It's less than two blocks."

Sawyer leaned over and opened the passenger door. "I thought I'd take the scenic route. Where are Scott and Susan?"

"In the yard. They wanted to run through the sprinkler." The temperature was in the low eighties for the second day in a row, and the kids loved it.

"Grab your swimsuit and a towel, and I'll take you and the kids to my favorite swimming hole," Sawyer suggested.

Abbey brightened. "You're on."

Scott and Susan came racing toward the truck when Sawyer pulled up in front of the yard.

"Say, kids, want to go swimming?"

"Can Eagle Catcher come, too?"

"Sure. Hop in the back," Sawyer told them.

Abbey hurried into the house and slipped out of her clothes and into her swimming suit. She almost hadn't packed it with the move. She threw on some shorts and a T-shirt, then grabbed towels and clothes for the children.

Sawyer drove out to the airfield and loaded them into a plane. He explained that this type landed on both land and water. It was a tight squeeze with kids and dog, but they managed. The kids thought it was great fun.

"How far is this swimming hole of yours?" Abbey asked once they'd taxied off the runway and were in the air.

"Far enough for the kids to appreciate it when we arrive."

From the air, there seemed to be a huge number of lakes. She did remember reading that there were—how many lakes? A lot—in Alaska, but knowing a geographical fact sure hadn't prepared her for actually seeing it. Above the sound of the engine, Sawyer explained that he was taking them to an all-around favorite spot of his. Not only was the swimming great, the fishing was good, too.

It must have been an hour, perhaps longer, before Abbey realized they were descending. She cast an anxious look at Sawyer before the plane glided gracefully onto the smooth water.

Once the engines had slowed, Sawyer steered the aircraft toward the shore.

"Does anyone know we're here?" she asked.

"I left a note for Duke."

"But—"

"Trust me," he urged. "I wouldn't take Scott and Susan anyplace where they wouldn't be perfectly safe." He patted her hand. "You, too."

"The kids have had only a few swimming lessons, but they're not afraid of the water." The lake was so clear Abbey could see the bottom. Near the shore, where Sawyer stopped, the lake appeared to be only three or four feet deep.

Various shrubs grew along the shoreline. Abbey recognized wild rose bushes and knew that in a month or so they'd be crowded with small, vibrantly pink flowers. It was easy to imagine the beauty they'd add to this already beautiful scene.

The minute they could step out of the plane, Scott and Susan were splashing about in the shallows. "It's cold, Mom," Scott shouted, grinning at her, his teeth chattering. "Wow, and does it ever feel good!"

"It's lovely," she agreed, dipping in one foot. "What's the name of the lake, Sawyer?" She was thinking she'd look for it on a map once they returned to Hard Luck.

Sawyer shrugged. "There are three million lakes in Alaska. They don't all have names. Let's call it . . . Abbey Lake."

"Abbey Lake!" Susan laughed.

"I like it," Abbey said, playing along. "It has a nice sound."

"Can we go in deeper now?" Scott asked. "I wanna swim."

"Hold your horses, son," Sawyer told him and tugged his shirt out of his waistband. He was undressed and down to his swimming trunks in almost no time; it took Abbey a little longer. Soon Sawyer and the two children were in waist-deep water and Scott and Susan were taking turns swimming short distances.

Abbey sat on the edge of the pontoon and dangled her feet in the water. It felt cold, but wonderfully invigorating.

"Come on, Mom! The water's great once you get used to it," Scott assured her.

"I think she might need some help getting wet," Sawyer teased.

"No. . . no! I'm fine." She saw the first splash coming in enough time to cover her face. But her defenses were hopeless against the concerted efforts of the other three. Within seconds she was drenched. "All right, you guys, this is war. The men against the women."

For a short while, pandemonium reigned. Abbey and Susan might have done more damage if they hadn't been laughing so hard. Abbey stumbled out of the water and onto the shore.

A few minutes later, Sawyer joined her. He wiped his wet face with his forearm, then sat down next to her on the sun-warmed sand. He kept his gaze trained on the children, who continued to wage war and fun.

"This was a fantastic idea," she said, wringing out her hair. "Thank you for thinking of us."

"I've been doing a lot of that recently," he said in a low voice. "Thinking of you," he clarified. "I feel my brother and I misled you about Hard Luck."

"I was the one who made the decision to come. I knew what I was getting into before I came. It's true the housing situation is a problem, but at the time you didn't know about the children."

"I wanted you to leave when you first came."

"I know," she said unevenly. His determination to be rid of her still rankled.

He glanced at her, his eyes intense. "I don't feel that way any longer."

"I'm glad," she whispered, finding it hard to keep the emotion out of her voice. She sighed softly, thinking how fortunate she was to have met Sawyer. He was wonderful with her children—wonderful with her. *To* her.

He looked away abruptly, as if the conversation had grown more personal than he'd intended. "When will the library open?"

"Funny you should ask. I had several inquiries this afternoon. I was thinking I'd place an Open sign on the door first thing in the morning."

"Great," he said, but it seemed to her that his response lacked enthusiasm.

Scott trotted out of the water and stood before them.

With some relief, Abbey turned her attention to her son.

"I was just watching you," he said, directing the comment to Sawyer, "and it looked like you wanted to kiss my mother." He grinned, scrubbing the water from his eyes with both hands. "You can if you want to," he announced, then raced back into the lake.

CHAPTER SEVEN

AT NINE O'CLOCK the following morning Abbey printed a huge Open sign and posted it outside the library. It didn't take long to get her first customer.

At five past nine, John Henderson ambled in, hands in his pockets. He was tall and husky, his boyish good looks set off by a thatch of honey-colored hair.

"Good morning," she said in a friendly tone.

"'Mornin'," he returned almost shyly. "It's a right pretty day, isn't it?"

"Sure is," Abbey agreed. The weather was unseasonably warm this year, she'd been told.

John wandered around the library scanning the rows of books.

"Is there anything I can help you find?" Abbey asked, eager to be of assistance.

"Yup."

"What do you like to read?"

"Romances," John said.

His choice surprised her, but she didn't let it show. Romances were generally considered women's fiction, but that didn't mean a man couldn't enjoy them.

"I need something that'll teach me the proper way to tell a woman I think she looks even prettier than a shiny new Cessna."

"I see." She suspected it would take more than a romance novel to help him in that area.

"I want to be able to tell her how pretty I think she is, but I need to know how to say it without riling her. Every time I try to talk to a woman, all I seem to do is make her mad. Last time I tried, I didn't do so well."

Abbey walked over to the bookcases and pretended to survey several titles while she thought over the situation.

"It's important I learn to talk to a certain woman right," John continued, "'cause another man's got a head start on the rest of us." His voice tightened. "But that's not important now, all things being equal, if you know what I mean."

Abbey didn't, but feared an explanation would only confuse her further. "You might look down this row," she finally advised, directing him to books on etiquette and social behavior.

"Thanks," John said, grinning widely.

Abbey returned to her desk. No sooner had she sat down when Ralph Ferris, another of Sawyer's bush pilots, casually strolled in. He paused when he noticed John. The two men glared at each other.

"What are you doing here?" Ralph demanded.

"What does it look like?"

"I've never seen you read a book before!"

"Well, I can start, can't I?" John glanced nervously toward Abbey. "I have as much right to be here as you."

"Is there something I can help you find?" Abbey asked the new man.

"I notice you shaved," Ralph taunted under his breath. "Good grief, what kind of after-shave did you use? It smells worse than skunk cabbage."

"I borrowed yours," John muttered.

The two men engaged in a staring match, then each attempted to force the other away from the bookcase. Bemused, Abbey watched Ralph butt his shoulder against John's. She saw John retaliate, jabbing the point of his elbow into Ralph's side. "If you two are going to fight, I'd prefer you didn't do it in the library," she admonished in her sternest librarian's voice.

The men scowled at each other, then rushed to stand in front of her desk. John spoke first. "Abbey, would it be all right if I stopped off at your house this evening?"

"How about dinner?" Ralph said quickly before she could answer. "Ben's cooking up one of his specials—caribou stroganoff."

"Dinner?" Abbey repeated, not knowing what to say.

Before she could respond, Pete Livengood marched into the room. His hair was dampened down as if he'd recently stepped out of the shower. He carried a heart-shaped box.

"Chocolates," the two pilots said together. They sounded furious—and chagrined—as if they'd been outmaneuvered.

"Women like that sort of thing," Abbey heard one whisper to the other.

"Where the hell are we going to get chocolates?"

"I've got an extra can of bug spray. Do you think she might like that?"

IT WAS TURNING into one of the most unproductive days Sawyer had ever spent.

His men had invented one excuse after another to delay their routine flights. He didn't need anyone to tell him they'd gone to the library, and they weren't interested in checking out a book, either.

Sawyer found himself increasingly impatient and ill-tempered. He refused to ask any of the men, but his curiosity made him incapable of concentrating. What was happening at that damned library? And how was Abbey reacting to attention from other men? The prospect of her being with someone else made him crazy.

Restlessly he stood in front of the office's only mirror, wondering if he should shave off his beard. He'd never asked Abbey how she felt about it. Although he'd worn a beard for more than ten years, he'd be willing to remove it if she asked.

He ran a hand along his face, then returned to his desk, slouching in the seat.

John had returned from the library first, clutching an old edition of Emily Post and a couple of paperback romances. Sawyer found him intently reading one of the love stories during his coffee break. He watched as John scanned a page or two, then set the book aside and stared into space. He seemed to be mulling over an important matter.

Ralph had dropped by the library early that morning, too. He'd come back sporting a book on the history of aircraft, which he proudly showed to Sawyer.

"I understand another woman's coming this week," Ralph stated, lingering inside the office. He glared at John accusingly.

"That's right," Sawyer answered absently, reading over a flight schedule before handing it to Ralph.

"I'd like to ride along."

"You already have a flight on Friday."

Ralph lifted one shoulder in a shrug. "Duke'll take it for me. He owes me one."

Sawyer didn't hesitate long. If two of the most woman-hungry of his men vied for Allison Reynolds, maybe they'd leave Abbey alone. So he agreed—with one stipulation. Duke had to willingly consent to the change in plans. Sawyer refused to arbitrate in a conflict over this, he told Ralph, and didn't want to hear another word about it. The other man's face fell as he walked out of the office and toward the airfield.

The day dragged by, with every single pilot somehow managing to visit the library. The minute Sawyer was free, he hurried there himself. He knew something was wrong the minute he stepped inside.

Abbey sat at the desk, and when the door opened, her head snapped up. Her eyes narrowed, she slapped a book shut. After observing the loving way she'd handled the books earlier, that action surprised him.

"Good afternoon," he said warmly.

No smile. No greeting.

He missed the warm way her eyes lit up whenever they met. He missed her smile.

He tried again. "How's your day going?"

Silence.

"Is, uh, something wrong?"

"Tell me," she said in tones as cold as a glacier, "exactly why was I hired?"

"Why were you hired?" he repeated slowly, not understanding her anger, let alone her question. "Hard Luck needed a librarian to organize a lending library."

"And that was the *only* reason?"

"Yes."

"Oh, really?" she spat out, her eyes blazing.

"Abbey, what's wrong?"

She stormed to her feet and folded her arms. The fire in her eyes was hot enough to scorch him from ten feet away. "All your talk about me breaking the spirit of the agreement! I can't believe I fell for that. You had me believing you were upset because I hadn't told you about Scott and Susan. Well, everything's clear to me now."

"That's settled and done with. No one blamed you—it was as much our fault for not asking."

Abbey shook her head, but Sawyer wasn't sure what she meant. It did seem to him, though, that she was close to ᴸears. The realization shook him. He stepped toward her, but stopped short of taking her in his arms.

"Stay away from me," she demanded.

"Abbey, please—"

"It wasn't a librarian you wanted," she said in a surprisingly calm voice. "You and your men were looking for—" she paused as if she didn't know how to continue "—entertainment."

"Entertainment?"

"I don't know how I could have been so *stupid*. The ad practically came right out and said it. Lonely men! You weren't interested in my library skills, were you? No wonder everyone was so upset when I arrived with children."

"That's not true," he flared. He did value her professional skills—and he didn't want her dating *or* "entertaining" any other man. Today, with every unattached male in Hard Luck visiting the library, had made that very clear to him.

"If the men in town are so lonely, why didn't you just advertise for wives?" she went on. "That's what everyone else does, isn't it?"

"Wives? We wanted women, but we didn't want to have to marry them."

Abbey's mouth fell open. "Oh. That makes it all right, then."

"We offered you a house and land, remember."

"In exchange for what?"

His temper was rising. "Not what you seem to think. We offered jobs, too, you'll notice."

"*Invented* jobs, you mean."

"All right, we *could* have organized the library with volunteers. But there was a reason for coming up with jobs, too."

"I'd be glad to hear it."

"Well, for one thing, no one wanted to be responsible for supporting a bunch of women."

"Is that what you think marriage is?" she flared.

"Damn right."

Abbey swallowed tightly. "You've told me everything I need to know." Her voice broke on the last word, and Sawyer felt shaken.

He tensed, knowing he'd botched this entire conversation. He tried to think of some way to explain the situation to her—without making things worse.

"It's lonely up here, Abbey. If you want to fault us for feeling like that, then go ahead. I was losing pilots left and right. Christian and I had to do *something* to keep them happy, and the only thing we could come up with was, uh, importing a few women." He knew that hadn't been the best way to put it, but he plunged on. "We wanted female companionship without the problems of marriage. We—"

"In other words, you wanted these 'imported' women to relieve the boredom." She closed her eyes as if he'd confirmed her worst fears.

"Did something happen to you today?" he asked, clenching his fists. "If anyone offended you, I'll personally see to it that he apologizes."

"*You've* offended me!" she cried.

"Why? Because I didn't offer to marry you? One woman's already tried to lure me into that trap."

"Trap?"

"I'm not going to marry you, Abbey, so if that's what you want, you'd better get this straight, right here and now. I brought you here so you'd be friends with a few of my men." Too late he realized how that must sound. "You know what I mean."

"I know *exactly* what you mean."

Sawyer could see that Abbey was in no mood to be reasonable. She'd already made up her mind, and nothing he said would change it. "We'll settle this later," he said gruffly.

She didn't respond.

Sawyer had to force himself to leave the library. He started down the walk, paused and started back, then stopped again. Damn, this was a mess. He hated leaving unfinished business.

Scott rode down the street on Ronny Gold's bicycle and pulled to a stop beside him. "Hi, Sawyer!" he said enthusiastically.

Sawyer's gaze was locked on the library door. "Hiya, Scott."

"How's it going?"

"Great," Sawyer lied.

"Ronny let me ride his bike. I'll sure be glad when mine gets here. How much longer do you think it'll take the shippers to haul our stuff to Hard Luck?"

Sawyer's eyes reluctantly drifted from the library to the boy. It seemed heartless to tell him that the truck wouldn't make it to town any time this summer.

"You miss your bike, do you?"

"It'd be neat if I had it, because then Ronny and I could ride together."

"I've still got an old bike from when I was a kid. I think it's in the storage shed. Would you like me to see if I can find it for you?"

Scott's eyes lit up. "Gee, that'd be great!"

"I'll go look for it right away," Sawyer promised, eager for an opportunity to prove himself a family friend, instead of the fiend Abbey thought him. He really didn't understand what had upset her so much. Good grief, what did she think when she answered the advertisement?

It took some doing to locate the old bicycle, which was tucked in the back of the shed behind twenty years of accumulations. Old as it was, the bike wasn't in bad shape.

Sawyer hosed it off in the front yard. When he finished the task, he happened to look up—and saw Abbey walking home.

He straightened, standing in the middle of his yard, the hose in his hand dripping water. He stared at her. With every bone, every muscle, every cell in his body, he ached to know what he'd done that was so wrong. More important, he needed to know how he could fix it.

Without even a glance in his direction, Abbey disappeared into the house. Not long afterward Scott approached him, frowning.

"The old bike doesn't look like much, does it?" Sawyer said, drying off the padded seat and chrome fender with an old T-shirt. "But I think once I get her cleaned up a bit and give the chain a shot or two of oil, it'll be fine."

"No, the bike looks great," Scott said, his sudden smile brimming with pleasure. But some of his enthusiasm faded when he looked over his shoulder. "I have to get home."

"If you wait a few minutes I'll have the bike ready for you."

"I think I better get home."

Sawyer looked over at his brother's house. "Your mother seems upset about something."

"I'll say," Scott muttered. "She's *real* upset."

Sawyer's gaze lingered on the front door, and the ache inside him intensified. He wouldn't rest until he'd settled this business with Abbey. "Maybe I should try to talk to her."

"Not now, I wouldn't," the boy advised.

Sawyer realized—with some embarrassment—how inept he was at dealing with women. Inept enough to accept advice from a nine-year-old boy. Still, if Scott thought it best to wait, he would.

"You'd think she'd be happy," Scott said with a long sigh. "Grandma and Grandpa kept telling her she should go out on dates, but Mom never showed much interest. She went out sometimes, but not very often. Now she's all upset because some guy asked her to dinner."

"Who?" Sawyer demanded before he could censor the question. "Never mind, Scott, that isn't any of my business."

"Well, Grandma wants her to marry again. I heard them talking once, and Grandma was telling my mom that it's wrong to let one bad experience sour her on marriage. She said there were lots of good men in this world and that Mom would find one of 'em, if she tried. Do you think my mom should get married again?"

Marriage wasn't a subject Sawyer felt comfortable discussing. "I...I wouldn't know."

"Mom's never said anything to us kids, but I think she gets lonely sometimes. Did you know Mr. Livengood asked her to marry him today?"

"Pete? What the bloody hell?" A fierce, possessive anger consumed Sawyer. He threw down the hose and was halfway out of his yard before he realized that he couldn't very well wring the bastard's neck. No matter what his feelings toward Abbey, Sawyer had no right to be angry. If Pete wanted to propose to her, that was his prerogative. He himself had no say in the matter.

"Scott!" Abbey had come out onto the porch to call her son. Sawyer might as well have been invisible for all the attention she paid him. "Dinnertime."

"In a minute, Mom."

"Now," she insisted.

"You'd better go," Sawyer advised. "I'll bring the bike over after dinner."

"Okay." He raced across the street, stopping when he reached the other side. "Sawyer," he called, "don't worry. I think Mom still likes you best."

Unfortunately the boy's opinion was damn little comfort.

ABBEY COULDN'T EAT; the food stuck in her throat. It was as if she were attempting to swallow gravel. The baked salmon certainly felt that way in the pit of her stomach.

Scott and Susan had never seemed more talkative, but she found it difficult to respond to their comments and questions.

"Sawyer said I could use his bike until mine arrives," Scott said, glancing expectantly at Abbey.

She'd been such a fool. It had taken her virtually the whole day to realize what was happening. Every unmarried man in town—most of them, anyway—had made a point of visiting the library, and it wasn't to check out books. No, it had more to do with checking out the librarian.

The newspaper ad had claimed there were lonely men in Hard Luck, but that wasn't the reason she'd applied. Not at all! Good thing, too, according to Sawyer.

"Don't you think that's neat of him to lend me his bike?" he asked.

Abbey had to think about the question before she could answer it. "Very nice."

"Did Mr. Livengood really ask you to marry him?" Susan piped up, her dark eyes wide with curiosity.

"Would you like some more rice?" Abbey asked, intent on changing the subject. The last thing she wanted to do was discuss the miserable details of her day.

"He said he was real serious," Scott said. "I overheard him telling Mrs. Inman that he wanted to get his bid in before anyone else."

Abbey groaned silently. How many more proposals would she have to endure? Apparently Sawyer was the only man in Hard Luck who *wasn't* interested in marriage. His ridiculous comment about her trying to lure him into the trap of marriage continued to rankle. As if she'd even *consider* such a thing.

"Are you going to marry him?" Susan asked.

"Of course not. I barely know Mr. Livengood."

"I think you should marry Sawyer, instead," Susan said thoughtfully. "Do Scott and I get to choose a new husband for you? 'Cause if we do, I bet Scott'd want Sawyer, too."

"I'm not marrying Sawyer O'Halloran," Abbey said, obviously with more vehemence than she'd intended, because both children gave her odd, confused looks.

"Why not?" Scott asked. "I think he's neat."

"He told us a bedtime story and took us swimming and named a lake after you, Mom. Don't you think he'd be a good husband?"

Abbey's shoulders sagged. "Let's not talk about Sawyer right now, okay?"

Scott and Susan accepted her suggestion without comment, for which Abbey was grateful. Both began to chatter about their new friends and their plans and Eagle Catcher and what they'd done that day.

It amazed her how well her children had adjusted to life in a tiny community. A town that lacked the amenities and resources they were used to. She'd been certain they'd find plenty of reasons to miss Seattle. They hadn't, even though they'd left behind their friends, their grandparents, their whole lives.

So had she.

After dinner Abbey was sitting alone at the kitchen table, drinking coffee and mulling over the woeful events of her day, when the doorbell rang. She answered it to find Sawyer standing on the stoop. Her heart thumped wildly.

His eyes held hers for so long it took her a minute to realize he had the bike Scott had mentioned at his side.

"Wait here and I'll get Scott," she said without emotion.

A muscle worked in his jaw. "I brought the bike over for Scott, but it's you I want to talk to." Nothing showed in his eyes, but she felt the power of the emotions he held under tight rein.

The same emotions churned inside her.

"Abbey, for God's sake, tell me what happened today."

"You mean other than two invitations to dinner and a marriage proposal? Oh, I nearly forgot—I was invited to inspect one pilot's fishing flies."

Sawyer closed his eyes. "That'd be John."

"Right. John. There were gifts, too."

The muscle in his jaw jerked again. "Gifts?"

"A bit of inducement, I suspect."

"I apologize for the behavior of my men. If you want, I'll drag every one of them down here to apologize."

"That's not what I want," she said coldly.

He heard the phone ring then, and with unconcealed relief, Abbey went to answer it.

SAWYER TOOK the mail run into Fairbanks himself. He found he could think more clearly when he was in the air. The roar of the plane's engines drowned out everything but the thoughts whirling inside his head.

He'd heard there were only two laws a pilot needed to concern himself with. The law of gravity and the law of averages. Whoever had said that hadn't taken into account the laws of nature—of physical attraction between a man and a woman.

Abbey confused him. Never had he been this attracted to a woman. The few kisses they'd shared had knocked him for a sensual wallop. It wasn't hard to imagine what the loving would be like between them.

He wanted her. Yet a saint couldn't fault him for the way he'd behaved toward her.

Frustration gnawed at him, eating away at his confidence. Granted, he hadn't been completely in favor of Christian's plan, but he didn't think it was unethical or unfair. It wasn't a question of false pretenses, at all. He didn't want to force anyone, man *or* woman, into a relationship. Not everyone wanted to become romantically involved; it was a personal decision. This way there was no pressure, but for the life of him, he couldn't make Abbey understand that. Offering women jobs, instead of marriage, meant everyone had a choice when it came to romance. Surely that was as much to the women's benefit as the men's!

The mere thought of her accusations infuriated him. His mouth thinned. He'd noticed it hadn't taken her long to bring up the subject of marriage.

Did he want to marry her? Did he love her?

Somehow Sawyer found it easier not only to think but to confront his emotions at thirteen thousand feet. What did he know about love? Damn little, he decided. From his earliest memories, his parents had been at odds. Somehow, he suspected, his parents had genuinely cared for each other, but in every other way theirs had been a bad match. Bringing his mother from the sophistication of London, England, to a primitive little community like Hard Luck couldn't have helped, either. Ellen had returned to England with Christian when Sawyer was thirteen. He'd never forgotten the desolate look on his father's face when the plane took off with his mother and youngest brother aboard.

It was the one and only time Sawyer could ever remember his father getting drunk. And he realized now, as an adult, that it was regret he'd seen in David's eyes.

Sawyer was well aware, as was Charles, when their father had started seeing Catherine Fletcher. He often wondered if David would have filed for divorce had Ellen not returned.

At first everything was better. His parents had decided to make a new start, and for a while, life in the O'Halloran household was smoother, and more pleasant than it had ever been. Sawyer hadn't realized how much he'd missed his youngest brother and his mother. At fourteen he hadn't understood the nature of his parents' relationship; all he knew was that he and his brothers were happy. Ellen had come back. They were a family again.

Unfortunately it didn't last. Everything changed abruptly, and his mother moved out of their master bedroom. To the best of Sawyer's knowledge, Ellen and David never slept in the same room again. Later, after the lodge was built, they didn't even sleep in the same house.

No one needed to tell Sawyer why this had happened. His mother had learned about David's affair with Catherine. No one needed to tell him how she'd found out, either. Catherine had taken a good deal of pleasure in breaking his mother's heart, destroying the tentative beginnings of happiness.

Sawyer had never understood why his parents didn't divorce. In the end, it was almost as if they'd *looked* for ways to make each other miserable.

No, his parents hadn't taught him about love. Nor had he learned much about it in the years since.

Until Abbey...

His mind filled with thoughts of her and Scott and Susan. If she was so distraught about her agreement to work in Hard Luck, he decided, then he'd release her from any obligation, real or imagined. She was free to go. He'd personally escort her and the children to Fairbanks and see them off, no worse for wear.

His heart beat high in his throat at the possibility of losing Abbey.

But if Sawyer admitted he loved her, he'd have to make a decision, and he wasn't ready for that either. Hell, they'd met less than two weeks ago. One thing was certain, though—he couldn't imagine Hard Luck without her now.

WHEN SAWYER RETURNED later that afternoon, he found Scott riding the old bicycle at the airfield. He spotted Eagle Catcher first and smiled to himself as he taxied the Cessna over to the hangar.

"You sure do fly good," Scott told him when he climbed down from the cockpit.

"Thank you, Scott."

"Are you going to take me up with you like you said?"

"Yeah, someday."

The boy's face fell. "That's what you said last time."

Sawyer remembered how much he'd disliked being put off when he was a kid. "You're right, Scott. I did say you could fly with me. Let's check the schedule."

"You mean it?"

"Yes, but we'll have to ask your mother's permission first."

Scott kicked the dirt with the toe of his sneaker. "I don't think you're her favorite person right now."

"She's still mad, is she?"

"Yup. She told Mr. Livengood she wasn't interested in marrying him. He looked like he was real disappointed, but you know what? I think he would've been surprised if she said yes."

"Maybe I should talk to her." Or try, although heaven knew he'd done that often enough.

"I wouldn't," the boy advised.

"Well, have you got any other ideas, then?" Sawyer needed all the help he could get, and he'd resigned himself to asking a nine-year-old boy for advice.

"The other guys brought her dumb gifts. Mom doesn't care about bug spray. She doesn't like mosquitoes, but we've gotten real good at keeping them away."

"Okay, I won't give her any bug spray. Can you think of anything she'd like?"

"Sure," Scott said, brightening. "She likes long baths with those smelly things that melt."

"Smelly things that melt?"

"Bath-oil beads," Scott said. "If you can get her those, she'd probably be willing to listen to you."

It was worth a try. He'd hit a drugstore next trip into Fairbanks. He walked into the office and held the door open for Scott to follow. Everyone had left for the day, which suited Sawyer fine.

He sat down at his desk; Scott sat in the opposite chair. Leaning back, Sawyer propped his feet against the corner and linked his hands behind his head. Scott imitated his actions, his knobby elbows sticking out like miniature moose antlers from the sides of his head.

A knock sounded at the door, and Susan stuck her head inside. Her smile widened when she found Sawyer and Scott. "I saw your bike outside," she told her brother. "Mom wants you."

"What for?" he asked.

"She needs you to help her carry some stuff home from the library."

"Okay," Scott said. He released a long-suffering sigh.

"Want me to come with you?" Sawyer offered. He didn't think Abbey would appreciate it, but then he hadn't seen her all day. Maybe, just maybe, she'd missed him as much as he'd missed her, and they could put this unpleasantness behind them.

"It's all right," Scott assured him. "I can handle it." He started toward the door.

"I appreciate the advice, Scott. Next run I make into Fairbanks, I'll buy plenty of those smelly bath things for your mom."

"Uh, Sawyer." Scott's face broke into a wide grin. "There's something else you could do."

"What's that?"

Scott and Susan exchanged looks.

"You could always marry my mom," the boy said. "Of the guys who've proposed so far, we like you the best."

CHAPTER EIGHT

So PETE LIVENGOOD wasn't the only one who'd popped the question, Sawyer mused darkly. Scott and Susan had said as much, and they were in a position to know. It infuriated him that the men in this community, men he thought he knew, would make such asses of themselves over the first woman to arrive. These were the very men who'd insisted all they wanted was a little female companionship. Yet the minute Abbey set foot in town, they were stumbling all over themselves to see which of them could marry her first.

Great, just great.

What bothered him even more were his own confused feelings for Abbey. He didn't want any of the other men in town pestering her—offering her gifts, dinner dates, marriage proposals. No, if anyone was going to do those things, he wanted it to be him. He just wasn't sure about the marriage part; he *was* sure about wanting to see Abbey. On an exclusive basis.

There, he'd owned up to it. But from the looks she'd given him lately, she'd rather go out with a rattlesnake than with him.

He sulked for a few minutes before leaving the office. He wondered if Mitch Harris had taken a liking to Abbey, too. Mitch barely knew Abbey, but then, that hadn't stopped Pete from proposing. Mitch, a widower, was a decent sort, and Sawyer knew Chrissy Harris and Susan had been palling around together; he hoped that wouldn't give Mitch an unfair advantage.

There were a number of other unmarried men in town. Ben Hamilton, for one. The owner of the Hard Luck Café was around the same age as Pete Livengood, and Sawyer considered him a good friend. But that didn't mean Ben didn't have eyes in his head. Abbey was a beautiful woman, and Sawyer could well understand why any man would be attracted to her.

There was no telling how many had lined up to offer Abbey their hearts and their homes. Not that he had a right to complain. It was more than he'd done. And a whole lot more than he intended to do.

Marriage was a lifetime commitment. Make that a life sentence. In his experience, marriage meant the death of love; it had sure killed whatever his parents had started out with. Well, he wouldn't let it happen to him. No, sirree. He was shocked and frustrated that the men of Hard Luck took their freedom so lightly.

As he continued his unsatisfying reflections, Sawyer strolled over to Ben's. It was too early for the dinner crowd, such as it was, and too late for lunch. The café was empty.

Sawyer slid onto the stool and uprighted a mug.

Almost immediately, Ben appeared from the kitchen and reached for the coffeepot. "What's eating you?"

Sawyer smiled to himself, amused and rather impressed that the cook could read him so easily. "How'd you know something's bothering me?"

"You came in for coffee, right?"

"Right."

"You got a pot at your office, same as I do here. I know I'm a good-lookin' cuss, but I don't think you're willing to pay a buck-fifty for a cup of coffee unless you need to talk. What's up?"

"It's that obvious?"

"Yeah." Ben picked up the empty sugar canister and re-filled it.

Sawyer wasn't sure where to start. He didn't want to let on that what he'd really come to learn was whether Ben had proposed to Abbey, along with everyone else in town.

"Let me help you out," Ben said when he'd finished with the sugar canister. "A man doesn't wear that damned-if-you-do damned-if-you-don't look smeared across his face unless a woman's involved. Is it Abbey?"

"Yeah." Sawyer couldn't see any reason to deny it. "Pete Livengood proposed to her." He raised the coffee mug to his mouth and studied Ben's reaction through the rising steam. The cook gave nothing away.

"So I heard."

"Apparently a few other men in town had the same idea."

Ben chuckled and brushed the sugar from his palms. "Someone else being interested in Abbey upsets you?"

That was putting it mildly. "Well, you could say I'm concerned," Sawyer admitted grudgingly.

Ben leaned against the counter and seemed to be waiting for him to continue.

"I know what you're going to say," Sawyer said before Ben could prod him. "You want to know what's holding me back. If I'm so worried Abbey'll marry someone else, why don't I propose myself? For a number of very good reasons, if you must know," he said, raising his voice. "Damn good reasons. First and foremost, I refuse to be forced into this. A man doesn't offer marriage lightly, or at least he shouldn't." He was thinking of Pete and the others. "Another thing. I won't have any woman dictating to me what I should and shouldn't do with my life."

Ben's face creased with a smug look. "Why are you yelling at me?"

Sawyer shut his eyes for a moment and shook his head helplessly. "The hell if I know." Once again, he couldn't help thinking about his own parents and how miserable they'd been together. Abbey had already been married once. Badly burned, too, as far as he could tell.

The cocky smile left Ben's face. "Maybe what you need to think about is if you love her."

That debate had been going on inside him all day. "I don't know what I feel," he hurled out.

"What about her kids?"

Some of the tension eased from him. "I'm crazy about those two. Scott and Susan are great."

Ben studied him as if seeing Sawyer in a whole new light. "You didn't think you'd ever really fall for a woman, did you? The fact is, before Abbey and her children got here, you thought you were happy."

"I am happy," Sawyer insisted.

"Sure you are," Ben muttered. Chuckling to himself, he returned to the kitchen.

"I'm damn happy," Sawyer shouted after him.

"Right," Ben called back. The old coot seemed highly amused. "You're so happy you're crying in your coffee, afraid Abbey Sutherland's going to marry someone other than you. Careful, Sawyer, she just might, and then what'll you do?"

Sawyer slapped a handful of coins down on the counter and left.

ABBEY INSERTED a card into the catalog and reached for the next one. This "low-tech" approach to librarianship was a far cry from the computerized system she was used to, she reflected, but for the moment, it was manageable. She glanced up as the door opened and Pearl Inman poked her head in. "Are you coming down to the airfield?" she asked.

"John Henderson's due back any time with Allison Reynolds."

"Give me a minute."

"I don't know about you, but I'm eager to meet this young woman," Pearl said, stepping into the library to wait. "Ben baked up a cake to welcome her. I just hope the men don't make fools of themselves the way they did when you arrived."

Abbey's heart fluttered with a mixture of dread and excitement as she pulled on her sweater and headed out the door. She was eager to meet Allison, eager to have another woman move to Hard Luck. If she remembered correctly, Allison was the woman Christian had mentioned the night he'd phoned—his dinner date.

It was inevitable that she'd run into Sawyer at the airfield; avoiding him in a town the size of Hard Luck was going to be impossible. Nor did she wish to. She'd been angry and upset the last time they spoke. She wasn't accustomed to a lot of attention from men; it flustered and alarmed her. Then Sawyer had arrived, and without intending to, he'd made everything worse. What upset her most was the way he'd insinuated she was hoping to trap him into marriage.

Despite what Sawyer may have thought, she *wasn't* planning to remarry. When she'd applied for the job, she'd done so because that was what she needed—a job. Alaska had sounded adventuresome, and small-town life had strongly appealed to her. One thing was certain, she hadn't come to "be friendly" with a bunch of love-starved men.

Unfortunately, once her children learned that Pete Livengood had proposed to her, they'd jumped on the bandwagon. Not that they wanted her to marry Pete. Oh, no, they were campaigning for Sawyer. Both Scott and Susan made sure they casually dropped his name at every opportunity. It was Sawyer this and Sawyer that, until she was sick of hearing about the man. Abbey didn't have the heart to tell them he was the last man she'd marry—even if he asked her. Not with that attitude of his. He'd live the rest of his days believing she'd tricked him into the arrangement.

The day was overcast and cool, a contrast to the warm sunshine the area had enjoyed all week. Shivering a little, she walked beside Pearl toward the airfield.

Half the town stood there waiting for the plane's arrival. Scott pulled up next to her on Sawyer's old bicycle, shading his eyes as he gazed into the sky.

"What's the big deal?" he asked.

"Sawyer's new secretary's arriving."

"Does she have any kids my age?"

The possibility amused Abbey. She wondered what Sawyer would do if another woman arrived on his doorstep with a family in tow.

"Probably not," she said.

"Are the men going to want to marry her too?"

"Maybe."

"Will Sawyer?"

"I wouldn't know about that," she answered again, more emphatically this time.

"I'd rather *you* married Sawyer," her son persisted. "Susan and me like him a whole lot, and he likes us."

"Scott, please!"

"But if he might marry this new lady, then don't you think you should do something about it?"

"No," she said in her sternest voice, praying no one was listening in on their conversation.

"I hear the plane," Pearl shouted.

Abbey squinted into the hazy skies. She could hear the buzz of an approaching aircraft, but wasn't able to see anything just yet. She recalled the excitement she'd felt when she'd first approached Hard Luck and looked down to find so large a welcoming committee.

The plane appeared over the horizon and slowly descended toward the dirt runway. Once it had taxied to a stop, Duke Porter hurried over and lowered the steps.

A minute later, a woman dressed in a hot-pink silk jumpsuit slowly moved down the steps. Like royalty, Abbey thought.

Allison Reynolds was beautiful, she realized with a small pang of jealousy. Knock-your-eyes-out gorgeous. Long legs that seemed to reach all the way to her earlobes, a more-than-ample bosom and a body that would stop New York City traffic. Allison gave a beauty-queen wave and the smile she bestowed on the crowd of welcomers was bright enough to create a glare.

Abbey was convinced every man present had to wipe the drool off his chin. Until that moment, she'd avoided looking for Sawyer, but now she scanned the crowd, seeking him out. She found him, his intense blue eyes glued to the latest arrival with undeniable interest. Just like the others.

Her heart chilled as she admitted to herself that he really wasn't any different. Disillusioned—and determined to ignore it—she squared her shoulders and looked away.

Lonely men, indeed. Well, they got what they wanted with Allison Reynolds. Thank heaven.

Just as they had when Abbey and the kids arrived, everyone assembled at the Hard Luck Café for introductions. Allison Reynolds was ushered inside and seated while the town put forth its best effort to impress her.

Abbey stood back and waited for a quiet moment to welcome the latest arrival. From her position by the wall, she had a clear view of the newcomer. Abbey sincerely hoped she and Allison would be friends. At the moment she could do with a friend.

"I'd like to talk to you."

Abbey started, then turned to discover Sawyer standing next to her. "Do you always sneak up behind people?" she asked in an angry whisper.

"Only when I'm desperate." He leaned one shoulder against the wall and crossed his arms. "It's Mitch Harris, isn't it?"

"What is?"

"The other man who proposed."

"That's none of your business."

"I'm making it my business. Was it Mitch?" he growled in a low whisper. Then not giving her time to answer, he asked again. "What about Ben Hamilton? I wouldn't put it past the old goat. He probably did it just to rile me." He sighed sharply. "Damn fool, it worked."

"As I said earlier, none of this concerns you." If there'd been anywhere to move, Abbey would have moved, but the café was packed. Why on earth would Sawyer choose this precise moment to talk to her?

"You aren't marrying any of them."

"I beg your pardon?"

"I'm serious, Abbey. Call me a male chauvinist pig or whatever else you want, but if you're so keen on finding a husband, then I'll marry you myself." His voice was harsh.

"You'll marry me yourself?" she asked, incredulous. "How generous of you. How benevolent!"

"I mean it," he said.

"Tell me, Sawyer, why would you do anything so...so drastic?" Mingled with her anger was a pain that cut deep, despite her disenchantment with Sawyer. This was exactly the type of behavior she'd come to expect from him—yet she was disappointed.

Her question appeared to hit its mark. His face tightened, and the muscle in his jaw leapt. Unable to bear listening to any more, Abbey walked out of the café. She'd introduce herself to Allison later.

She hadn't gone only a few feet when she heard the sound of the screen door slam behind her. Quickening her steps, she hurried away.

"Abbey, wait."

Sawyer.

It didn't take him long to catch up with her. "For heaven's sake, will you stop long enough to listen to me?"

Her throat was clogged with tears, making it impossible to answer him. He steered her onto the airfield and into a nearby hangar, then turned to face her. His outstretched arms cupped her shoulder.

Abbey kept her face averted, praying he'd say whatever he intended to say so she could leave.

"Why do I want to marry you?" He repeated her question, and it sounded as if he felt as confused as she did.

"You don't want me," she accused. "All you care about is making sure I don't accept anyone else's proposal. Your ridiculous male pride couldn't take that! Well, if you thought you were appeasing me with this insulting offer of marriage, you're dead wrong."

"I do want you," he argued, pulling her into his arms.

Her heart stopped, then jerked back into life as he directed her mouth to his. The kiss was long and thorough. Groaning softly, he kissed her again, hungrily this time. Her lips parted, and she slid her arms tightly around his hard waist.

They engaged in a series of warm, moist kisses that gained in intensity. His tongue met hers and explored the softness of her mouth. He drew her closer until the full lengths of their bodies were pressed together. She felt the rise and fall of his chest and knew her own breathing was as labored.

Suddenly, looking stunned, he dragged his mouth away from hers. He dropped his hands, releasing her, and stepped back.

Abbey studied him for a moment. "Don't look so worried, Sawyer," she said with wounded dignity. "I'm not going to accept your proposal." She spun on her heel and walked away, grateful he chose not to follow her.

AS IT HAPPENED, Abbey got a chance to talk to Allison Reynolds later that same afternoon. They met in the road outside the library. After a few minutes' conversation, it was apparent—at least to Abbey—that the other woman had no intention of staying in Hard Luck and probably never had.

"You're Abbey," Allison said, smiling. "Christian mentioned that he'd hired you." She crossed her arms and swatted at a mosquito. "Can we talk?" Allison asked, doing a poor imitation of Joan Rivers. "I'm dying to find out what's happened to you since you arrived." Allison glanced both ways, then lowered her voice conspiratorially. "Are you going to stay?"

"I plan to. So far, I love Alaska."

"But it's summer," Allison said as if this was something Abbey hadn't yet figured out. "I don't think anyone was serious about us staying all winter, do you? I mean, this is the *Arctic*. I don't go anywhere in the winter where there isn't a hot tub."

"I've never lived through an Arctic winter before, so I can't say, but I do know I intend to try."

"You do?" The new secretary of Midnight Sons made it sound as though Abbey was making a serious mistake. "Anyway, I can't talk long. I'm supposed to meet Ralph and Pearl, and they're going to drive me out to the cabin. I've never owned a home of my own. Christian said it's a quaint little place. I can hardly wait to see it. But I do hope someone finds a way to get the rest of my luggage up here soon. They seemed to think I could pack everything I own in three suitcases."

Before Abbey could describe her own experience, Allison was gone. Actually Abbey was just as glad not to be around when Allison viewed her "quaint" new home.

The rest of the afternoon passed slowly, the main attraction in town being the vivacious and beautiful Allison Reynolds and not the newly opened Hard Luck Lending Library.

Pearl Inman was watering her cabbage plants when Abbey strolled past on her way home.

"What a sorry disappointment Allison Reynolds is," Pearl Inman muttered. "That Christian's got mush for brains. I can't imagine what he was thinking when he hired her."

Abbey grinned. "Himself most likely."

"That girl got a free trip to Alaska—which was all she wanted," Pearl said with a disgruntled look. "Makes me downright angry to think of the way everyone's been looking forward to meeting her."

"She might change her mind and stay."

"It'd be a mistake if she did. Allison Reynolds is the type who causes more problems than she solves. My guess is she'll be out of here before the week's up."

Personally Abbey agreed with Pearl.

"I saw you and Sawyer talking. I'm glad to hear you decided to put that boy out of his misery."

Abbey wasn't aware that her troubles with Sawyer were common knowledge. "If Sawyer O'Halloran's miserable, he has no one but himself to blame."

"Isn't that the way it is with most folks?"

Abbey had no argument there.

"As for what happened to you this week, with the men and all, well—" Pearl sighed "—I have to say I blame Sawyer for that."

"So do I," Abbey said. And if he assumed he could make everything better by tossing her a marriage proposal, he was mistaken.

"The men wouldn't have come at you like a herd of buffalo if Sawyer hadn't tried to keep you for himself," Pearl continued. "Way I hear it, some of them were up in arms because of all the rules and restrictions he put on them."

"Rules?"

"He didn't want anyone pestering you. However, he didn't include himself in that. But this is the only time in his life I've ever seen Sawyer take advantage of a situation. You know," the older woman said thoughtfully, "I don't think he realized he was doing it. His intentions were to help you and the children get settled. I know for a fact he never intended to fall in love with you."

Abbey looked away to hide her sudden tears. Sawyer *didn't* love her. His proposal told her that much. He was afraid she'd accept someone else, so he'd put his offer on the table. Only a day earlier, he'd vehemently insisted he wasn't marrying anyone.

"I'll see you later, Pearl," Abbey managed.

Her friend cast her a look of concern. "You all right, sweetie?"

Abbey nodded, but she wasn't. What truly frightened her was that she'd fallen in love with Sawyer. Once before, she'd proved what a poor judge of character she was when it came to men. She'd left the marriage broken, her confidence destroyed. She blinked back the tears that stung her eyes, feeling a strange new desolation.

Abbey was nearly home when she noticed a truck driving toward her. She knew almost everyone in town by now, and stared at the unfamiliar yet somewhat familiar face as the truck slowed to a stop.

"Hello," the driver said.

"Hello," she responded, sniffling slightly.

"I'm Charles O'Halloran."

"Abbey Sutherland," she whispered.

Charles frowned. "Do you mind telling me what's going on around here?"

SAWYER SAT in his office, rolling a pen between his palms. Every time he talked to Abbey he made matters worse. It started when he saw her standing on the airfield waiting for Allison Reynolds's arrival. His heart had actually ached at the sight of her. Even now he didn't know what he'd done that was so terrible, and Abbey didn't seem to want to tell him.

A man had his pride, but he'd been willing to swallow it one more time, so he'd followed her into Ben's place. Then, before he could stop himself, he was drilling her about other men, acting like a lunatic. He'd never been jealous in his life, and he didn't know how to handle it. John, Pete, Duke, Ralph, Mitch and the others were his friends. Or had been.

The office door opened and without a word of warning, in stepped his oldest brother. "Charles!" Sawyer bolted to his feet. "Damn, but it's good to see you. When'd you get in?"

"About an hour ago." Charlie slipped the backpack from his shoulders and set it aside.

Charles looked good—tanned and healthy. He was a leaner, taller version of Sawyer, people often said.

Walking over to the coffeepot, Charles poured himself a mug.

Sawyer knew his brother well enough to realize something was troubling him. "You got a problem?"

His brother sighed and sipped at the coffee. "Can you tell me how you happened to let your brain go all soggy in the space of a few weeks?"

Sawyer laughed. "So you heard about the women."

"That's exactly what I'm talking about."

"We flew them up. And there's more coming."

"We?"

"Christian and me. Midnight Sons."

"To live?"

Sawyer nodded, the humor leaving him. Just as he'd expected, Charles didn't think much of their scheme. "We came up with the idea of offering them those old cabins Dad built plus twenty acres of land. In exchange, they have to agree to live and work in Hard Luck for a year." As he spoke, Sawyer realized how ludicrous their idea must sound to their levelheaded older brother. It had to him at first, too, but his arguments had grown less convincing after Abbey's arrival.

"The women are supposed to *live* in those old cabins?" Charles asked incredulously.

"We cleaned them out, Charlie. They're actually quite...clean."

With unexpected violence, Charles slammed down his mug. "Have you two gone nuts?"

"No. We did what we thought was necessary to help the community grow." Sawyer was aware that he sounded stiff and pompous.

"It wasn't Hard Luck you were thinking about when you advertised for women," Charles countered sharply. "You were thinking of yourselves."

"We were losing pilots left and right," Sawyer snapped. "Phil's gone, and we were about to lose Ralph and John as well. The men were willing to stay if we could bring in a few women."

"How many do you have coming?"

"I don't know," Sawyer confessed, trying to suppress his own anger. "Christian took care of that end of it."

"Was it Christian who sent up the beauty queen, or are you the one responsible for that?"

"Beauty queen? Oh, you mean Allison. No, she was Christian's idea. Okay, she probably won't work out. We're bound to have a few failures, but that's the law of averages. Some women are going to be able to adjust and become part of our community. Others won't."

"Allison Reynolds wants out of the deal. Claims she was sold a false bill of goods. I talked to her myself—ran into her at Ben's."

"Fine. I told you—I didn't expect her to last. I'll arrange for her flight back to Seattle. All I have to do is tell Christian, and he can send up another secretary. From what I understand, there are plenty of applicants."

"Which brings up something else neither of you seemed to trouble yourself with. The media."

Sawyer had gotten a number of inquiries, but he'd steadfastly refused to give interviews. Way up here, he felt relatively safe from the press.

"You aren't so naive as to think the press doesn't know, are you?" Charles asked.

"Of course they know," Sawyer answered. "But they didn't hear about it from me. Before long, it'll be old news and everyone'll leave us alone."

"For your information," Charles said tersely, "I read about your scheme in the Anchorage newspaper while I was in Valdez."

"Okay, so the news is out," Sawyer muttered, unconcerned. He had more important things to worry about than some unwanted press.

"What do you think'll happen when they learn you've already got a failure on your hands? These women don't know anything about Alaska. They left everything they had and flew up here, thinking God knows what and expecting something far different than what they were promised."

"Okay, Allison was a failure, and frankly I blame Christian for that. But Abbey Sutherland's one of the best things that's ever happened to Hard Luck. She's already got the library organized and in operation."

"Abbey Sutherland's the one living in Christian's house, right?"

"Yes." He didn't think now was the time to admit the mistake they'd made on the application form. Nor did he want Charles to know he'd contacted Catherine Fletcher's daughter about the use of Catherine's home for Abbey and her children.

"It seems you've misjudged the situation with her."

Sawyer's head snapped up. "Just what the hell do you mean by that?"

"She isn't staying."

Sawyer's gaze narrowed. "Who told you that?"

"Abbey herself."

Sawyer felt as if he'd had the wind knocked out of him. It took a long moment for him to be able to think clearly. "You met Abbey?"

Charles nodded.

"She's staying," Sawyer said, not waiting to hear his brother's argument.

"Sawyer, damn it, will you listen to reason?" Charles shouted.

"I don't give a damn what Allison Reynolds decides," he told his brother between gritted teeth. "But Abbey and her kids are staying."

Charles groaned. "She has children, too?"

Sawyer rushed toward the door.

"Where are you going?" his brother demanded.

"To see Abbey."

He made the trek between the office and Christian's place in record time. He arrived, breathless with anger and exertion, at her front door, his shoulders heaving. Instead of knocking, he hammered his fist against the door.

Abbey answered it and stared at him through the screen.

"You aren't leaving." His voice was a harsh whisper.

"Sawyer," Charles shouted from behind him. "What do you think you're doing?" He leapt up the porch steps. "We've already talked about you going back to Seattle, remember?" he said to Abbey, lowering his voice.

Abbey stood on the other side of the screen door, her hand over her mouth.

It was all Sawyer could do not to rip the door off its hinges and haul her into his arms. "Abbey, listen, I—"

"Sawyer, leave the poor woman alone," Charles broke in.

Sawyer whirled around. "Stay out of this, Charles. This has nothing to do with you and everything to do with me." The two men glared at each other.

"Abbey," Charles said, looking past his brother. "Like I said, you don't have to live in Hard Luck if you don't want to. I'll personally pay for your tickets back to Seattle."

His brother's words felt like a knife between his shoulder blades.

"I said I'd marry you," Sawyer reminded her, his voice raised. "Isn't that what you want?"

"No. It isn't what I want." With that, she started to close the front door.

"Abbey," he cried, frantic to talk some sense into her.

The door closed. He battled back the temptation to open it and follow her inside.

The realization hit him that he was going to lose her, and there wasn't anything he could do about it. The last time he'd experienced such hopelessness had been the last afternoon he'd spent with his father.

CHAPTER NINE

"WHAT'S FOR DINNER?" Scott asked on his way through the kitchen. He didn't give Abbey time to answer. "Can we have macaroni and cheese? Not from a box, but the kind you bake in the oven?"

"Sure." Abbey made sure she kept her back to her son in an attempt to disguise how upset she was. For the second time that day, her eyes were brimming with tears.

All the contradictory emotions that had buffeted her for the past few days had reduced her to a kind of helpless inertia. For the first time since her divorce, Abbey had allowed herself to fall in love—with a man who didn't know how to love, who didn't *want* to love.

Allison Reynolds was sure to leave. She was the smart one, Abbey thought bitterly. The one who willingly owned up to a mistake and took measures to correct it. That was what Abbey should have done—only earlier, much earlier, before her heart became so completely involved.

She'd made one devastating mistake by marrying Dick. She'd known it almost immediately, but instead of admitting her error, she'd tried to make the best of a bad situation. She'd had to struggle for years to get her life back in shape.

Then, a few weeks ago, she'd begun to dream again, to hope, to believe that it was possible to find happiness with a man. Her illusions had been painfully shattered, one by one. It'd all started when she realized her position as Hard

Luck's librarian had been a ruse—she'd been brought to Alaska to provide "female companionship" to a bunch of love-starved bush pilots.

Sawyer didn't want her to leave, that much he'd made clear. She wasn't sure why, though, and knew he wasn't, either. He was resisting whatever feelings he had for her, resenting them. He'd offered to marry her, but from the way he'd proposed, he seemed to consider marriage to Abbey some kind of punishment.

"Can Eagle Catcher come inside while we eat?" Scott asked, breaking into her thoughts.

Despite her misery, Abbey smiled. "You know the answer to that."

"But, Mom," Scott said in a singsong voice, "I was hoping you'd change your mind. Eagle Catcher may be a dog on the outside, but on the inside he's a regular guy."

Her son seemed intent on lingering in the kitchen. He opened the refrigerator and took out a pitcher of juice to pour himself a tall glass. "I saw you talking to some strange man earlier. In a truck." Scott waited as if he expected her to fill him in on the details. When she didn't, he added, "I thought it was Sawyer at first, but he doesn't have a beard."

"That was Charles O'Halloran, Sawyer's brother."

"Oh." Scott pulled out a chair and sat down at the table. He didn't say anything for a long moment. Finally he asked, "Are you all right, Mom?"

"Sure I am," she said with forced enthusiasm. "Where's Susan?"

"She's playing with Chrissy Harris, like always. Do you want me to get her?"

"In a bit."

Scott finished off the juice, then headed for the back door. "Don't be late for dinner," she called after him.

"I won't, especially if we're having macaroni and cheese."

Her mind preoccupied with her own problems, Abbey thought it was quite an accomplishment that she didn't burn dinner. In spite of her earlier resolve to stay, in spite of the fact that she'd invested everything she had in moving here, Abbey came to a decision. By the time her children trooped in, the table was set and she was ready to address the unpleasant task of telling them they'd be leaving Hard Luck. Abbey knew Scott and Susan weren't going to like it.

They sat down at the dinner table together, and Abbey waited until they were halfway through the meal before broaching the subject. "I understand Allison Reynolds has decided she doesn't want to stay," she mentioned casually. "She's flying out first thing in the morning."

"The new lady looked like a ditz to me," Scott commented between mouthfuls of macaroni and cheese.

"She's real pretty," Susan said.

"She's dumb."

"Scott!" Abbey interjected.

"Well, she is. Anyone who didn't like this place after we threw a party for her is more than dumb, she's *rude.*"

"Allison looked nice, though," Susan said thoughtfully. She stopped eating and studied Abbey.

Scott seemed far more concerned about stuffing down as much macaroni and cheese as possible, as quickly as possible. If Abbey had been a betting woman, she'd have said Eagle Catcher was on the front porch waiting for him.

"You know," Abbey said carefully. "I'm not so sure it's the right place for us, either."

"You gotta be kidding!" Scott cried. "I like it here. I was kinda worried if I'd find new friends when we first got here. But it's neat being the new kid on the block. Everyone wants to be my friend, and now that Sawyer's let me have his old bike, it's just like being back home."

"There's no ice-cream man," Susan said, gesturing with her fork. She continued to study Abbey.

"There's no place for us to live, either. When Mr. O'Halloran offered me the job, I didn't tell him I had a family."

"Why can't we stay right here?" Susan wanted to know. "This is a nice house."

"Because this house belongs to Sawyer's brother Christian," Scott answered for her. "Sawyer told me that he was going to phone some old lady who used to live in town but doesn't anymore. He thinks we should be able to rent her house. We don't have a problem, Mom. Sawyer's taking care of everything."

"It's not just the living arrangements," Abbey went on. "The trucking company can only take our furniture as far as Fairbanks. There's no way to get it to Hard Luck until winter."

"I can wait," Scott volunteered.

"Me, too," Susan agreed.

"What about our supplies for winter?" she asked.

Both children stared at her as if she were speaking another language. "What does everyone else do?" Scott asked.

"They buy enough supplies to last them a year at a time. Best as I can figure, that'd be nearly five thousand dollars for the three of us. I can't afford that."

"Can't you get a loan?" Susan suggested.

"No. I didn't know any of this, and now, well, it just makes sense for us to leave."

"But Sawyer—"

"Please," she said, cutting Scott off. Abbey sighed deeply. The last person she wanted to hear about was Sawyer. But she could see that it was going to take more than excuses to convince her family they had to move away from Hard Luck.

"I'm beginning to think we made a mistake in leaving Seattle," she whispered, barely able to look across the table at the children.

"A mistake? No way!"

"We like it here!" Susan protested.

"It's been a wonderful experience," Abbey said, "but it's time to stand back and assess the situation. We have some important decisions to make."

"You made the decision a long time ago," Scott insisted. "Don't you remember what you told us? You said that no matter what, we'd give it a year, and then we'd decide what we wanted to do. It isn't even a full month yet and you're already talking about quitting."

"There are things you don't understand," Abbey said. No one had told her that when she agreed to move to Alaska, she'd be putting her heart at risk. She'd never have taken the gamble had she known the stakes were so high.

Over the past few weeks, she'd learned she could live without indoor plumbing. She could manage without electricity. She could even do without the luxury of a shopping mall close at hand. But she could not tolerate another man crushing her heart.

And Sawyer would.

Sawyer didn't know about love, didn't trust it. His parents' difficult marriage had left him wary and cautious; she wasn't much better.

She'd taken all the pain she could bear from one man. She wasn't giving Sawyer the opportunity to take over where Dick had left off. As cowardly as it was, she'd made up her mind to leave.

She didn't expect her son and daughter to understand or appreciate that, which made everything more difficult.

"You aren't serious about moving, are you, Mom?"

Abbey swallowed over the tightness in her throat and nodded.

"I thought you liked it here," Susan said.

Everyone stopped eating. Scott and Susan stared at her from across the table, their eyes huge and forlorn.

"It just isn't working out the way I figured," she told them brokenly.

"Is it because of Sawyer?" Scott asked.

Preferring not to lie, Abbey didn't answer him. "Since you both enjoy Alaska so much... I was thinking we could find a place in Fairbanks. Since that's where the truck's delivering our furniture, I thought we could rent a house and... and settle in before school starts again."

"I don't want to live in Fairbanks," Susan said emphatically. "I want to live here."

"I'm not leaving Eagle Catcher," Scott told her in a deceptively calm voice. From past experience, Abbey knew it wouldn't be easy to convince her son to change his mind.

"There'll be lots of dogs in Fairbanks."

"Why do we have to leave?" Susan wailed.

"Because... because we have to. Hard Luck is a wonderful town with lots of friendly people, but... but it hasn't worked out for us."

"Why not?" Scott pressed. "I thought you liked it here. Sawyer even named a lake after you, remember?"

There wasn't much she *didn't* remember about her times with Sawyer. The emotion that had hovered so close to the surface all day broke through, and hot, blistering tears filled her eyes.

"I'm so sorry..." Angry with herself for succumbing to this, Abbey swiped at her face and dragged a deep breath through her lungs, hoping it would relieve some of the tension.

"Why are you crying, Mommy?" Susan asked.

Abbey patted her daughter's shoulder and stood up to reach for a tissue.

"Is this because of Sawyer?" Scott demanded for the second time. "Is he the one who made you cry?"

"No. No!"

"You were mad at him earlier."

Abbey didn't need to be reminded of Sawyer's role in this drama. But ultimately she didn't blame him. If anyone was at fault, she was—for believing, for lowering her guard and falling in love again. For making herself vulnerable.

"Everyone says you should marry Sawyer," Susan put in. "If you did, would we still have to leave Hard Luck?"

"If you don't want to marry Sawyer," Scott said, "what about Pete? He's not as good-looking as Sawyer and he's kinda old, but he's real nice, even if he does wear his hair in a ponytail. We could live with him, and he's got more than enough supplies to last us all year."

"I'm not marrying anyone," Abbey insisted, laughing and crying simultaneously.

"But if you did want to marry someone, it'd be Sawyer, right?" Scott persisted, his eyes serious. "You really like him. I know you do, because Susan and me saw you kissing, and it looked like you both thought it was fun."

"We're friends," Abbey told her children. "But Sawyer doesn't love me and... Oh, I know you're disappointed. I am, too, but we have to move."

Neither of the children said anything.

Abbey sniffed. She wiped her nose with her tissue, then rested her hands on the back of the dining-room chair. The sooner they were gone the easier it would be, she decided. "Pack everything in your suitcases tonight. We're leaving first thing in the morning with Allison Reynolds."

SAWYER SAT ALONE at the dinner table, his meal untouched. When Charles returned to Hard Luck from one of his jaunts, the two brothers usually sat up and talked away most of the night.

Not this time.

Sawyer swore if he saw his older brother just then, he wouldn't be held accountable for what he said or did.

His own brother had turned traitor on him by offering to fly Abbey out of Hard Luck. Sawyer had hoped she'd have the common sense to realize she belonged right here with him. But apparently not.

Thanks to Charles's interference, his encouraging Abbey to leave, the two brothers had become involved in a heated exchange. They'd parted, furious with one another.

Even now Sawyer couldn't understand how the brother he'd have trusted with his life could do this to him. It was obvious that Charles didn't know a damn thing about falling in love. And even less about women.

Sawyer prayed that his older brother would experience—and soon—the intense frustration of loving a woman and being barricaded at every turn. And he *did* love her, damm it.

It was particularly disconcerting when one of those barricades came in the form of his own flesh and blood.

Not for the first time since meeting Abbey, Sawyer appreciated the dilemma his father had been in when his mother had announced she wanted a separation. Soon afterward, Ellen had packed her bags and returned to England with Christian.

Although he'd only been a young teenager at the time, Sawyer remembered the day his mother had left. Wordlessly his father had driven her to the airfield, watching as the plane disappeared.

Even now, Sawyer couldn't fully understand the dynamics of his parents' relationship. He'd realized for years that his mother was deeply unhappy. As a child, he'd known she wasn't like the other women in Hard Luck. She spoke with an accent and tended to keep to herself. As far as Sawyer knew, Pearl Inman had been her only friend. The other women had club meetings and volunteered at the school, but Ellen was never included.

In some ways she'd been an embarrassment to her son. He'd wanted her to be like his friends' mothers. All she ever seemed to care about were her books—and yet, ironically, it was those books that had brought Abbey to Hard Luck.

Like his father before him, Sawyer was going to walk down to the airfield come morning and watch the woman he loved disappear into the horizon.

Then, like his father, Sawyer strongly suspected he was going to get royally soused, if not falling-down drunk.

Pushing his untouched dinner plate aside, Sawyer stood. He walked into the living room and gazed longingly out the window. Abbey was directly across the street, but she might as well be on the other side of the world.

The urge to breach the distance and tell her everything that was in his heart was like a gnawing hunger that refused to go away. If there was the slightest chance she'd listen to him, he'd have done it.

From the corner of his eye, Sawyer watched Scott wheel his old bike toward his house. The boy threw the bike down, then kicked it hard enough to make Sawyer wince.

First the mother and now the boy. Exhaling a deep breath, Sawyer stepped resolutely to the front door and opened it. He walked onto the porch. "Is something wrong, son?"

"I'm not your son!" Scott shouted.

"What's wrong?"

Scott kicked the bicycle again. "You can have your dumb old bike back. I don't want it. It's stupid and I never liked it."

"Thank you for returning it," Sawyer said without emotion. Scott's display of pain and anger was unlike him. Wondering what—if anything—he should say, Sawyer walked down the steps. "Would you like to help me put it back in the storage shed?"

"No."

Sawyer stooped to pick up the bicycle. The moment he bent to retrieve it, he was attacked with fists and feet. The blows didn't hurt as much as surprise him.

"You made my mother cry!" Scott screamed. "Now we have to leave!"

Sawyer easily deflected the impact of the small fists and wild punches. Scott kicked him for all he was worth, his shoe connecting with Sawyer's shin a number of times.

In an effort to protect himself and Scott, Sawyer dropped the old bike and wrapped his arms around the youngster's shoulders. He knelt down on the grass in front of him. By now Scott was crying openly and his breath came in ragged gasps.

Sawyer held him tight, soaking in the boy's pain and thinking his own heart was about to break. Losing Abbey was bad enough. It seemed unfair that he'd lose the children, too.

In the short time they'd lived in Hard Luck, Scott and Susan had captured his heart. A day didn't seem right without Scott there to greet him and ask if he could get Eagle Catcher out of his pen. And Susan . . . With her wide grins and charming enthusiasm, she could always wrap his heart around her little finger.

"I'm sorry I made your mother cry," Sawyer whispered over and over, although he was sure the boy didn't hear him.

Sobbing, Scott buried his face in Sawyer's shoulder. Soon his thin arms were wrapped around Sawyer's neck and he clung to him as if he never wanted to let go. "Your bike isn't really stupid," he mumbled.

"I know."

"We have to pack everything back inside our suitcases," Scott said. "Mom told us at dinner that we're leaving in the morning."

"I know." He didn't bother to disguise his regret.

Scott's head jerked back and he stared at Sawyer through swollen eyes. "You do?"

Sawyer nodded.

"And you were just going to let us leave, without even a goodbye?"

"I was going to walk down to the field in the morning and see you off," Sawyer explained. *And then silently stand by and watch you fly away.* He had no choice. What else could he do?

"Susan and I don't want to leave."

Sawyer's heart lightened a little. Perhaps Abbey's children could succeed in talking sense into her where he'd failed so miserably. "Did you tell your mother that?"

Scott's eyes glistened with his recently shed tears. "That made her cry even more. I thought you cared about Mom and Susan and me."

"I do, Scott, more than you'll ever know."

Scott yanked himself free. "Then why does Mom want to move away so bad, and why are you letting her?"

"Because..." Sawyer struggled for the words. "Sometimes it isn't easy to explain, especially when you're just nine and—"

"I wouldn't understand it if I live to be as old as... as forty."

Sawyer smiled, despite himself. "I wish I understood it myself so I could explain it to you." He stroked the boy's hair. "Do you want to talk about it some more?"

"No," Scott said, and shook his head. Rubbing his eyes with the heel of his hand, he turned and ran in the opposite direction as fast as his legs would carry him.

Sawyer's heart contracted at the boy's distress. He wanted to follow Scott and swear that he'd do anything to convince Abbey to remain in Hard Luck. Anything. Instead, he remained standing on the front lawn, staring after her son. He hardly noticed that Mitch Harris was walking in his direction.

At Mitch's greeting, he raised a hand and smiled wanly. Presumably the public safety officer wasn't there on official business. In his calm, quiet way, Mitch was the most effective cop they'd ever had, but right now, Sawyer didn't need a cop.

"You certainly look down in the mouth," Mitch said, continuing toward him.

Sawyer kept his gaze trained on the house across the street. "Abbey's leaving," he said flatly.

"You're kidding, I hope. Her daughter and my Chrissy hit it off like gangbusters."

"I know."

"It's been great for Chrissy to have a friend her age," Mitch said, his eyes narrowed in concern. "Those two have been inseparable for the past month. What happened?"

"I'll be damned if I can figure it out." Sawyer massaged his forehead.

"I thought—or rather, I'd heard talk that you and Abbey had become . . . good friends."

"I thought we were friends, too. I guess I was wrong. She wants out of Hard Luck."

"Are you going to let her go?"

For pride's sake, Sawyer shrugged as if her coming or going was of little consequence to him. "It seems bringing women to town was nothing more than an expensive mistake."

"I'm sorry to hear about Abbey and her kids leaving, though," Mitch said. "Chrissy's going to miss Susan, and I suspect Hard Luck's going to miss having a librarian. Abbey would've done a good job if she'd decided to stay on. It's a shame, really."

Sawyer couldn't agree more.

"That's not our only problem," Sawyer said. He went back into the house and brought back a letter addressed to the school board from Margaret Simpson, the high-school teacher. "I received this in today's mail," he said and handed it to Mitch.

Mitch quickly scanned the letter's contents. "Margaret's decided not to teach next year, after all."

"That's what she says." She'd addressed the letter to Sawyer as president of the school board. He drew a deep breath. "It looks like we're going to be needing another teacher before the end of the summer. I'll be calling a board meeting later in the week."

"All right. It seems like a lot of bad news all at once doesn't it?"

Sawyer's gaze centered on the house across the street. "That it does," he murmured.

The two men shook hands, and Mitch left, walking across the street to Abbey's house. Sawyer had never been the nosy type, but he was decidedly curious to learn what Mitch intended to say.

Abbey answered the door. Although Sawyer couldn't hear the conversation, he guessed that Mitch was bidding her farewell. But whatever Mitch's business with Abbey, it didn't last long. Hoping he wasn't too obvious, Sawyer tried to sneak a look at her. It didn't work; she was back inside the house faster than a turtle retreating into its shell.

NEITHER OF THE CHILDREN had been particularly cooperative about going to bed. Since the sun still shone brightly at ten o'clock, it was difficult for them to go to sleep quickly. As usual, Abbey propped a board against the curtains to darken the room a little.

She was grateful when the talking quieted down. Sitting at the kitchen table with her feet on the opposite chair, she sipped from a glass of iced tea and mulled over her options.

Her suitcases were packed. So were the children's. They'd worked silently, together, not hiding their disappointment. It was such a contrast, Abbey thought, to their cheerful, excited chatter the night they'd packed to come here.

Before he'd gone to bed, Scott had told her he'd returned Sawyer's bike. Abbey had hugged her son and kissed the top of his head.

Fairbanks wouldn't be so bad, she'd tried to convince herself and the children. It was Alaska's second-largest city, and it would have all the comforts they'd left behind in Seattle.

No reaction.

She'd assured them they'd be settled in and ready long before school started. Even the reminder that Fairbanks was the world's mushing capital didn't seem to raise Scott's spirits. He was going to miss Sawyer's husky.

"Will I ever see Eagle Catcher again?" he'd asked.

"I . . . I don't know," Abbey told him sadly.

Although she knew she wouldn't sleep, she trudged down the hall to her bedroom. Out of habit, she stopped to check on Scott and Susan. Knowing they hadn't been asleep for long, she opened the door a crack and glanced inside.

Both had the covers pulled over their shoulders. Quietly she closed the door and slipped down the hall.

She got as far as the second bedroom when she paused. Something wasn't right. She hesitated, unable to identify exactly what it was. Retracing her steps, she returned to the bedroom, opening the door a bit wider this time.

Standing as she was, her silhouette against the opposite wall, Abbey could see nothing wrong. Tiptoeing farther into the room, she sat on the edge of Scott's bed.

It was then that she realized it wasn't her son in the bed at all, but a rolled-up blanket and a football helmet.

Abbey gasped, surged to her feet and tore back the covers.

Scott was missing.

She rushed over to the second bed and discovered that Susan was gone, too.

Abbey turned on the light and found an envelope leaning against the lamp on the nightstand. She reached for it, her fingers trembling so hard she could barely find the strength to open it.

Dear Mom,
We don't want to leave Hard Luck. You can go without Susan and me. Don't worry about us.

Love,
Scott and Susan

Abbey read through it four times before the realization began to sink in. Her children had run away.

She raced to the phone and instinctively dialed Sawyer's number. She felt so shaky she had to punch in the numbers twice.

"Hello."

At least he wasn't asleep. "It's Abbey. Is Eagle Catcher there?"

"You want to talk to my dog?"

"Don't be ridiculous. I want you to check his pen and tell me if he's inside. Please, Sawyer, this is important."

"I can tell you right now that he is," Sawyer grumbled. "I locked him inside no more than an hour ago."

"Please check."

"All right."

She heard the click as he set the phone down. Abbey closed her eyes and impatiently counted backward, starting at one hundred, while he left the house to check his backyard. She'd reached sixty-three by the time he got back.

"He's gone," Sawyer said breathlessly. "Abbey, are you okay? What's happened?"

"No, I'm not okay." Her heart felt like it was about to explode inside her chest. "Scott and Susan are gone."

Without a second's hesitation, Sawyer said, "I'll be right over."

"Please hurry," she whispered, but he'd already severed the connection.

CHAPTER TEN

"WHERE WOULD THEY GO?" Abbey demanded even before Sawyer was in the house. She handed him Scott's letter, which he read in a few seconds.

"I have no idea."

Abbey sank onto the sofa. Her legs were incapable of supporting her any longer. "This is all my fault."

"Blaming yourself isn't going to help find those kids. Think, Abbey! You know Scott and Susan. Where would they hide?"

Abbey buried her face in her hands as she tried to reason it out, but her mind refused to function. Every time she closed her eyes, all she could visualize was her two children out in the wilderness alone. Sawyer had repeatedly warned them about the dangers lurking on the tundra. He'd told them about his aunt, who had disappeared without a trace at the age of five....

No one had ever explicitly described the dangers of brown bears, but it was very real. The day after her arrival she'd learned how to operate a can of pepper spray to ward them off. Now her children, the life and breath of her soul, were alone and defenseless, possibly wandering around in the wild. Eagle Catcher could only do so much to protect them.

"I'll find them, Abbey," Sawyer promised. He knelt down in front of her and gripped her hands in both of his.

"I swear to you I won't stop searching until they're home and safe."

Instinctively Abbey reached for him. Despite their differences, despite the fact that she was walking out of his life in a few hours, she trusted Sawyer as she did no one else. He'd find her children or die in the attempt. She knew that.

His arms gripped her, and they clung to each other.

"Abbey, don't forget—they've obviously got the dog with them. That's a good thing. Stay here," he instructed. "I'll alert Mitch and we'll get a search team assembled."

She nodded, well aware that she wouldn't be of any help to them. But she didn't want to be here alone with her fears. Sawyer seemed to realize that, too.

"I'll ask Pearl Inman to come stay with you."

Her heart in her throat, Abbey walked with Sawyer to the front door. He raised his hand and gently touched her cheek. Then he was gone.

Abbey moved onto the porch and sat in the swing, nearly choking on her fears. Mosquitoes buzzed nearby, but she paid them no heed. Again and again, her mind went back to the conversation she'd had with the children earlier that evening.

They loved Hard Luck. And Eagle Catcher and Sawyer. Without a bit of trouble, they'd adjusted to their new lives in Alaska. Abbey had assumed it was too soon for any real attachments to form, but she'd been wrong.

Her son had bonded with Eagle Catcher. He'd become friends with Ronny Gold. Susan had struck up a friendship with Chrissy Harris. And she . . . well, she'd gone and done something really dangerous.

She'd fallen in love with Sawyer O'Halloran. She saw her actions with fresh clarity. Knowing she loved him frightened her so badly she'd decided to run. The fear of making another mistake had caused her to panic.

Pearl appeared on the top porch step. Caught up in her thoughts, Abbey didn't notice her right away.

"Abbey?"

"Oh, Pearl," she said in a broken whisper. "I'm so afraid."

The older woman sat down next to her and squeezed her shoulders. "Sawyer will find those kids, don't you worry."

"But they could be anywhere."

"Mark my words, they'll be found in short order. At least they were smart enough to take Eagle Catcher with them. He's a good dog, and he isn't going to let anything happen."

Abbey tried to relax, and despite Pearl's assurances, found it useless. The tension wouldn't ease until her children were home and safe.

"Come on," Pearl said, "let's make a pot of coffee and some sandwiches. The men are going to need them."

Abbey agreed to help, although she realized Pearl was just trying to get her mind off the children. She moved into the kitchen and began the preparations by rote.

"Are you sure you want to use that much coffee?" Pearl asked, looking up from the bread she was efficiently buttering.

Abbey saw that she'd filled the basket to overflowing. "No," she said, laughing nervously. "Perhaps you'd better make the coffee."

"Sure thing. Let me just finish this."

They sat at the kitchen table and listened to the hot water drip through the filter. The pot's gurgling seemed obscenely loud in the unnatural quiet of the house.

An hour passed, the longest of her life. Mitch stopped by the house and asked Abbey a number of questions about the kids.

When he left, Pearl poured her a cup of coffee.

"The kids were upset about leaving," Abbey confessed to her.

"You're leaving?" Pearl sounded shocked. "Whatever for?"

"Because... oh, I don't know, because nothing seems right anymore. I'm afraid, Pearl... I don't want to be in love. It scares me. And Sawyer... I would've thought it was impossible to insult a woman with a marriage proposal, but he managed it. He seems to think every woman wants to trap him!"

Pearl gently patted her hand. "If that's the case, he must feel very strongly about you, otherwise he'd never have asked you to be his wife."

Despite everything, Abbey smiled. "I think Sawyer's as confused as I am."

When the phone rang, it startled Abbey so much, she didn't know what to do. She sat paralyzed, unable to move or breathe or think.

Pearl picked up the receiver. "Yes, yes..." she said, nodding.

Abbey studied the older woman's face for any sign of news.

A moment later, Pearl held her hand over the mouth-piece. "It's Sawyer. He called to let you know they have two four-man teams searching the area. The first one just reported back. They didn't find any trace of the children. He wants to talk to you."

Abbey snatched the receiver. "Sawyer, what's happening?" She pleaded for news, any news.

"Nothing yet." How calm and confident he sounded. "Don't worry, we'll find them. Are you all right?"

"No!" she cried. "I want my children!"

"We'll find them, Abbey," he said again. "Don't worry."

She took a deep breath and tried to remain calm. "Is there any sign of Eagle Catcher?" she asked. If they found the dog, then surely the children would be close at hand.

"Not yet."

"Call me again soon, please. Even if you haven't found them. I need to know what's happening."

"I will," he promised.

Pearl poured Abbey another cup of coffee and brought it to her. She stared into the rising steam, trying to think.

Another hour dragged slowly by. Restless now, Abbey started to pace. This time when the phone rang, she leapt for it.

"Did you find them?" she blurted into the mouthpiece.

"Mom?"

"Scott, is that you?" Abbey asked, then burst into tears. The release of tension washed over her like...like the clear, clean waters of Abbey Lake.

"Don't cry, Mom. We're fine. I bet we're in a lot of trouble... Here, you better talk to Sawyer."

Abbey tried to control her emotions, but the relief was too great to do anything but give in to it. A moment later Sawyer was on the line.

"Abbey, it's me."

"Where were they?"

"We found them in the old lodge. They'd managed to make their way upstairs, where they were hiding. I found the three of them cuddled up together. Eagle Catcher was in the middle and they each had an arm around him."

"You mean to say they were that close to town all this time?"

Sawyer chuckled. "Yup. Eagle Catcher heard me calling him, but he wouldn't leave Scott and Susan's side."

"Remind me to kiss that dog." She laughed softly.

"I'd rather you kissed the dog's owner."

Abbey's laughter faded, and the tension returned.

"Never mind," Sawyer said, defeated. "It was only a suggestion. The important thing is, the kids are safe and sound. I'll be bringing them home."

"Thank you, Sawyer. Thank you!" She glanced over at Pearl as she replaced the telephone receiver. "They're fine," she said, wiping the tears from her face. Sawyer found them hiding in the lodge."

"Thank God," Pearl whispered.

"I do," Abbey responded.

"I don't imagine you'll be needing me here any longer." The older woman started toward the door, then stopped and turned. "I know it's none of my affair and I'm sticking my nose where it doesn't belong, but I'd rather hoped you'd stay on in Hard Luck. You don't need me to tell you what stubborn cusses men can be—and Sawyer's more stubborn than most. But his heart's in the right place."

Uncomfortable with the conversation, Abbey averted her gaze.

"We're gonna miss you and those young'uns," Pearl said sadly, "but you're the one making the decisions."

Abbey walked her to the door, then stood and waited on the porch for Sawyer to deliver her family. He arrived in his truck, along with his brother. When he opened the door, Scott and Susan came charging out of the cab, running straight to Abbey's outstretched arms.

Both children were talking at once, telling their version of what had happened and why. After she'd hugged and kissed them both, she glanced up to find Sawyer standing beside the truck, watching them. Charles remained inside the cab.

"It seems to me you've managed to cause a lot of trouble," she told the children sternly. "You'll both be writing letters of apology to each and every person who searched for you."

Scott hung his head and nodded. Susan did, too.

"I'm sorry, Mom," Scott said, "but we don't want to move to Fairbanks. We like it here."

"We'll discuss your reasons in the morning. We'll also discuss your punishment, and it's going to be more than writing the letters. Understand?"

They nodded again.

"Now go and take a bath, both of you—you're absolutely filthy. Then climb back into bed. We've got a busy day ahead of us in the morning."

"But, Mom—"

"Good night, Scott. Good night, Susan," she said pointedly.

With their heads hanging, the two youngsters made their way into the house.

Abbey looked at Sawyer. Drawing a deep breath, Abbey approached him. "Sawyer, I don't have the words to thank you properly," she said, wrapping her arms around her waist. She smiled hesitantly at him. Even now, the temptation to walk into his arms tempted her almost beyond endurance. It struck her as deeply significant that when she'd found her children missing, he was the person she'd instinctively turned to.

"I'm glad they're safe," Sawyer said. "That's what matters."

They stared at one another, neither saying a word or moving a step closer.

An eternity seemed to pass before Charles stuck his head outside the cab window and cleared his throat. "We'll be seeing you in the morning, right?"

Abbey looked from Sawyer to Charles. "In the morning," she said, then turned and walked away.

"YOU LOOK LIKE you could use a good, stiff drink," Charles said when Sawyer climbed back into the truck.

Sawyer's eyes were fixed on the front door of the house. It'd take a hell of a lot more than whiskey to cure what ailed him.

"I'll drive you back to your place," he said impassively. He tightened his hands around the steering wheel until his knuckles showed white.

"You're in love with her." Charles's voice was matter-of-fact.

"Is that so hard to believe?"

"You barely know the woman!"

Hot anger surged through Sawyer. "I know what I feel. I know that when Abbey and those two kids board the plane you're piloting tomorrow, they're taking a part of me with them."

"You're serious?"

"You're damn right I'm serious!" Sawyer snapped.

Charles didn't say anything until his brother pulled up in front of his house, which was at the other end of town near the lodge. "I was wrong to get involved."

It was of little comfort to have Charles admit it now.

"I sure don't think this scheme of yours and Christian's was one of your brighter moves, but you obviously really care for Abbey and those children."

His brother wouldn't understand how much he did care until he'd fallen in love himself. "That's putting it mildly."

"Are you going to let her leave?"

"What choice do I have?" Sawyer asked, frustration ringing in his voice. "I can't hold her hostage. I've tried talking to her, and that doesn't do any good. Mainly because every time I open my mouth to tell her how I feel, I end up insulting her. I get all tongue-tied and stupid."

Charles seemed to find Sawyer's confession amusing. He smiled.

"I've never...felt this way before," Sawyer said in his own defense, "and I'm telling you right now, watch out, because it's like getting hit with the worse case of flu you've ever had. Your turn's coming, big brother, so get that smug look off your face."

"No way," Charles insisted. "I don't want any part of that. Look what it's done to you."

"You think I wanted this? It just *happened*. Abbey arrived—and there I stood with my tongue hanging out."

Charles laughed outright. "How is it, little brother, that we've lived to the ripe old ages of thirty-three and thirty-five without falling in love?"

"And we were proud of it, weren't we, big brother?" Now it was Sawyer's turn to be amused. "Not anymore. When I met Abbey, I felt like I'd been sucker-punched. So I did everything I could think of to get rid of her."

"What made her decide to leave?"

"You mean other than my marriage proposal?"

Charles laughed. "So you scared her into it."

"I was serious, damn it. All right, maybe I didn't use fancy words and tell her the angels smiled on her the day she was born and drivel like that, but I meant what I said." He paused, as the regret sank in. "Maybe I could have been a bit more romantic about it, though."

"What'd you say to her?"

"Well—" Sawyer thought back to their conversation "—I don't exactly remember. We were at Ben's and there were a lot of people around, so I sort of stood next to her and said I didn't think it was a good idea for her to marry Pete or any of the other men who'd proposed."

"You mean to say she had more than one offer?"

"Yes." Sawyer's fingers threatened to dent the steering wheel. "Besides Pete, I think Ralph might've asked her, too."

"So you stood next to her at Ben's..."

"Right. We were welcoming Allison Reynolds, and basically I told Abbey that if she was so keen to get married she should've said something because I was willing to marry her."

Charles was strangely quiet. "That was it?"

Sawyer nodded.

"You didn't ask for my advice, but I'll give it to you, anyway. If I were you I'd ask again, and this time I'd use a few of those fancy words you frown on."

"I don't know that I can," Sawyer said sadly.

"Can you live with the alternative?" Charles asked.

"I don't know," he said. "I just don't know."

After dropping his brother off, Sawyer returned to his own place. He checked on Eagle Catcher, talking to the dog for a few minutes, then walked into the house. If felt strangely empty and silent. He fixed a drink and took it into his bedroom, where he spent some time studying the photographs of his parents that stood on the dresser.

Tugging his shirttail free, he undressed and readied for bed. It was going to be a long night. Lying on his back, hands cupping his head, he stared at the ceiling and tried to work on his options.

What he'd told his brother was true. When Abbey left Hard Luck she'd be taking part of him with her. He had to prove that to her. He just didn't know how.

He wasn't a man of words. He'd repeatedly shown that; he'd made a mess of things every time he opened his mouth. There *had* to be a way to show Abbey he loved her.

He hardly slept at all.

By six he was up and dressed again. He sat at the kitchen table, nursing his coffee, devising a plan.

He waited until eight, then gathered together what he needed. He walked purposefully across the street to Abbey's.

He hadn't even reached the front door when she opened it. She wore a pretty pink sweater and jeans, and she'd never looked more beautiful.

"Good morning," she said, and he realized how pale she was. Pale and miserable. As miserable as he was.

"'Morning."

"I know you're busy getting ready to leave, so I won't take any more of your time than necessary. I brought something over for Scott and Susan," he said. "And you."

"The children are still sleeping."

"It doesn't matter. I'll give what I have to you, and you can see that they get it later."

"Sawyer, I've been thinking and really there isn't any need—"

"Would it be all right if we sat down?" He motioned toward the swing.

Abbey sighed and perched on the swing's edge. Sawyer had the impression she'd rather avoid this last encounter. He didn't blame her.

They each sat on opposite sides, as if they were uncomfortable strangers. He handed her an envelope. "These are Eagle Catcher's registration papers. I'm giving him to Scott—it'll help make the transition easier. Once you're settled, let me know and I'll have him delivered."

"But he's *your* dog."

Sawyer's smile was sad. He wouldn't tell her that relinquishing the husky was more difficult than she'd ever know. "Those two belong together."

"But, Sawyer—"

"Please, Abbey, let me do this one thing."

She looked as if she wanted to argue with him, then bit her lower lip and nodded.

"Susan is a wonderful little girl," Sawyer said. "I thought long and hard about what I could give her." He reached inside his shirt pocket and withdrew a gold, heart-shaped locket. "This belonged to my grandmother." He opened the tiny clasp with difficulty. "The picture inside is of Emily, the daughter she lost who was never found. She gave it to me shortly before she died. I'd like you to keep it until Susan's old enough to wear it."

Tears welled in Abbey's eyes as he lowered the locket and chain into the palm of her hand. "Sawyer, I...I don't know what to say."

Sawyer's heart was heavy. "I have no other way of showing you how much I love you and Scott and Susan." He stood and reached into his pants pocket and took out an envelope containing two marbles, a bobby pin and several folded sheets of paper. He sat down, then retrieved a second envelope from his shirt pocket.

"The last things I have are for you." He gave her the bobby pin first. "This saved my life when I was sixteen. It's a long, involved story that I won't go into, but I was flying alone in the dead of winter and I had engine trouble. Had to make an emergency landing. This bobby pin was on the floor of the plane, and it helped me fix the problem so I could get back in the air and home. Otherwise I would've frozen to death. I saved the pin." He set it carefully aside.

Abbey smiled.

"The marbles were my two favorites as a kid. I was better than anyone, and these were the prize of my collection. Mom special-ordered them for me from a Sears catalog."

Abbey held the two marbles in her free hand.

He handed her the folded sheets of paper. "These are old and a bit yellow, but you should still be able to read them. The first is an essay I wrote when I was in junior high. I won a writing contest with it and got a letter of commendation from the governor. His letter's with the story."

Abbey used the back of her hand to wipe the tears from her face.

Sawyer withdrew a plain gold band from the second envelope. "This is my father's wedding ring." Sawyer held it up between two fingers. His heart clenched with pride and pain at the sight of it. "Since I was the one with Dad when he died, Charles and Christian thought I should have it. It's probably not worth much, but I treasure it." He leaned forward to place the ring in Abbey's hand and closed her fingers over it. Afraid he might have said more than he should, he stood up and awkwardly stuffed his hands in his pockets. "Goodbye, Abbey."

As he turned to leave, she called to him. "Sawyer."

He faced her.

"Why are you giving me these things?"

"The bobby pin and marbles and the essay and Dad's ring—they represent what I am. I can't go with you and I can't make you stay, so I'm giving you part of me to take when you leave."

He was halfway down the steps when he heard her whisper. "You might have said you loved me earlier."

He kept his back to her and answered, "I want to marry you. A man doesn't propose to a woman unless he loves her."

"He does if he's afraid some other man might beat him to the punch. He does if he's confused about what he really wants."

"I know what I want," Sawyer said, turning, and his eyes met hers.

"Do you, Sawyer?"

"I want to spend the rest of my life with you, right here in Hard Luck. I want to raise Scott and Susan as my own children, and if you and God are willing, I'd like another child or two."

They stood staring at each other, the depth of their emotions visible. Abbey's beautiful brown eyes glistened with tears. It demanded every bit of self-control Sawyer possessed not to crush her in his arms and kiss her senseless.

"But I can't have that," Sawyer said, "so I'm giving you the most valuable things I own to do with as you please." Having said that, he hurried down the remaining steps.

"If you walk away from me now, Sawyer O'Halloran, I swear I'll never forgive you."

He turned back around to find her standing on the top step, her arms open. The sweetest smile he'd ever seen lit her eyes, curved her mouth.

His heart came to a sudden standstill. Then he rushed back, throwing his arms around her waist, pulling her tight against him. He trembled with the shock of how good she felt. He kissed her gently at first, for fear of frightening her with the power of his need.

Abbey wrapped her arms around his neck and moaned. A stronger, more disciplined man might have been able to resist her, but not Sawyer. Not when he feared he'd never hold her and kiss her again. Not when he'd laid his heart and his life at her feet.

They kissed again, too hungry for one another to attempt restraint. It was as if all the barriers between them had disappeared.

When he could, Sawyer pulled his mouth from hers, inhaled deeply and buried his face in her neck. He prayed for the strength to stop; otherwise, he feared he'd end up making love to her right then and there. But Abbey drew his face to hers, and the kissing began all over again.

"I think you should marry me," he breathed between kisses.

"A woman prefers to be asked, Sawyer O'Halloran."

"Please, Abbey, if you have any feelings for me whatsoever, put me out of this misery and marry me."

"Are you asking me, or telling me?"

"Begging."

He felt the rush of air from Abbey's gentle laugh before she kissed him. The kiss was deep and shockingly thorough.

"Is that your answer?" he panted when she'd finished.

"Yes. But first you need to understand. I'm not very good at this wife thing. I've got one failure behind me, and, oh, Sawyer, I'm so afraid."

"Of what? Making another mistake?"

"No, not that. Not with you. I'm afraid . . . of so many things. Dick had several affairs, and when we divorced, he said . . . he said I'd never make a man happy."

"You make me happy. Did I ever tell you how much I love it when you smile?"

Abbey blushed. "I don't mean it like that. I don't know if I'll . . . satisfy you."

Sawyer threw back his head and laughed. "Oh, Abbey, just holding you gives me so much pleasure I can't even begin to imagine what it's going to be like in bed."

Sawyer could see that she was about to argue with him, so he guided her mouth to his and kissed her with all the love he had stored in his heart. He tasted her reluctance and her fear, then felt her weaken and give herself over to the kiss.

For the first time Sawyer understood the root of Abbey's fears. "You satisfy me," he whispered. "And tantalize me and torment me."

"Mom."

Sawyer looked past Abbey to find Scott and Susan in the doorway. They were both still in their pajamas, their young faces bright and wide-awake and eager.

"Good morning," Sawyer said. "I've got some great news for you."

"You do?" Susan asked.

"Your mother's agreed to marry me."

Scott looked mildly puzzled. "Already? Mom, I thought you said it would take awhile to work out the problems between you and Sawyer."

"Work out our problems?" Sawyer repeated. He was the one wearing the perplexed frown this time.

"The children and I talked after you found them last night," Abbey explained, and kissed the tip of his nose.

"We decided it would be a mistake for us to leave Hard Luck. Furthermore, we decided we're in love with you."

"You mean to say you weren't going to leave?"

Abbey's arms tightened around him. "Don't sound so disappointed."

"I'm not. It's just that...." He stiffened. "You might have said something earlier."

"I tried, but you wouldn't let me. Are you sorry now?"

"No," he said fervently. "Not in the least."

"Are you really going to marry us?" Susan wanted to know.

"Yup."

"When?" This was from Scott, who continued to look unsure.

Sawyer and Abbey exchanged glances. "Two weeks," Sawyer said, making the decision for them.

"Two weeks!" Abbey cried.

"I've been waiting thirty-three years for you, Abbey Sutherland, and I refuse to wait a minute longer. We'll do this as plain or as fancy as you want it. Ben can cater the wedding, and we'll open up the school gymnasium for the reception."

A truck pulled up on the street and the driver honked. "Looks like you two have everything settled," Charles called, leaning his elbow out the window.

"Yup."

"Guess you won't be needing me, then."

"Sawyer's going to marry Mom and us," Susan informed him with her wide, delightful grin.

"In two weeks," Scott added.

"So you're not letting any grass grow under your feet," Charles commented.

"Nope," Sawyer said.

"Is this a secret or can I spread the word?" Charles asked.

Abbey and Sawyer looked at each other and smiled. "Feel free," Sawyer told him.

Charles pounded the horn and stuck his head out the window and drove down the street shouting, "There's going to be a wedding in Hard Luck!"

"There's no changing your mind now, Sawyer O'Halloran."

"No fear of that," he whispered. "No fear at all."

* * * * *

Will Charles be the next Midnight Son to fall in love? Is there a woman who can change his mind about marriage?

Find out next month in The Marriage Risk, *the second book in Debbie Macomber's* **MIDNIGHT SONS.**

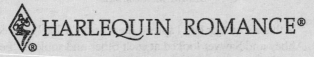

HARLEQUIN ROMANCE®

Coming Next Month

#3383 THE MARRIAGE RISK Debbie Macomber
The second book in Midnight Sons, a very special new six-book series
from this bestselling author.

Welcome to Hard Luck, Alaska. Population: 150—mostly men! Location:
north of the Arctic Circle. And meet the O'Halloran brothers, who run a
bush-plane service called Midnight Sons. They're also heading a campaign
to attract women to their town....

In *The Marriage Risk*, Charles O'Halloran, the oldest brother, finally
decides to take a chance on marriage. But there's something he doesn't
know about Lanni Caldwell, the woman he's fallen in love with—
something important.

#3384 CHARLOTTE'S COWBOY Jeanne Allan
Charlotte Darnelle wanted to make one thing clear—she was not a redhead.
She was a strawberry blonde, and any man who thought otherwise was in
deep trouble. Needless to say, rancher Matthew Thornton was in it up to
his Stetson!

#3385 SISTER SECRET Jessica Steele
Family Ties
Belvia had been trying to protect her painfully shy twin, Josy, from the
attentions of Latham Tavenner, and now he thought she was a loose
woman—deserving of his contempt! Belvia couldn't afford to alienate
him—the family firm badly needed his financial support. So how long
would it be before Latham took advantage...?

#3386 UNDERCOVER LOVER Heather Allison
Sealed with a Kiss
There was no room for sentiment in the newspaper business. And
certainly no room at all for the blistering attraction Kate Brandon felt for
Maxwell Hunter! The celebrated photographer might have come to her
rescue once, but she couldn't, wouldn't, fraternize with a man she was
competing with to get an exclusive picture. And as for falling in love...

MILLION DOLLAR SWEEPSTAKES (III)

No purchase necessary. To enter, follow the directions published. Method of entry may vary. For eligibility, entries must be received no later than March 31, 1996. No liability is assumed for printing errors, lost, late or misdirected entries. Odds of winning are determined by the number of eligible entries distributed and received. Prizewinners will be determined no later than June 30, 1996.

Sweepstakes open to residents of the U.S. (except Puerto Rico), Canada, Europe and Taiwan who are 18 years of age or older. All applicable laws and regulations apply. Sweepstakes offer void wherever prohibited by law. Values of all prizes are in U.S. currency. This sweepstakes is presented by Torstar Corp., its subsidiaries and affiliates, in conjunction with book, merchandise and/or product offerings. For a copy of the Official Rules send a self-addressed, stamped envelope (WA residents need not affix return postage) to: MILLION DOLLAR SWEEPSTAKES (III) Rules, P.O. Box 4573, Blair, NE 68009, USA.

EXTRA BONUS PRIZE DRAWING

No purchase necessary. The Extra Bonus Prize will be awarded in a random drawing to be conducted no later than 5/30/96 from among all entries received. To qualify, entries must be received by 3/31/96 and comply with published directions. Drawing open to residents of the U.S. (except Puerto Rico), Canada, Europe and Taiwan who are 18 years of age or older. All applicable laws and regulations apply; offer void wherever prohibited by law. Odds of winning are dependent upon number of eligibile entries received. Prize is valued in U.S. currency. The offer is presented by Torstar Corp., its subsidiaries and affiliates in conjunction with book, merchandise and/or product offering. For a copy of the Official Rules governing this sweepstakes, send a self-addressed, stamped envelope (WA residents need not affix return postage) to: Extra Bonus Prize Drawing Rules, P.O. Box 4590, Blair, NE 68009, USA.

Become a Privileged Woman,
You'll be entitled to all these Free Benefits. And Free Gifts, too.

To thank you for buying our books, we've designed an exclusive FREE program called *PAGES & PRIVILEGES™*. You can enroll with just one Proof of Purchase, and get the kind of luxuries that, until now, you could only read about.

Big HOTEL DISCOUNTS

A privileged woman stays in the finest hotels. And so can you—at up to 60% off! Imagine standing in a hotel check-in line and watching as the guest in front of you pays $150 for the same room that's only costing you $60. Your *Pages & Privileges* discounts are good at Sheraton, Marriott, Best Western, Hyatt and thousands of other fine hotels all over the U.S., Canada and Europe.

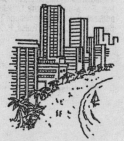

Free DISCOUNT TRAVEL SERVICE

A privileged woman is always jetting to romantic places. When you fly, just make one phone call for the lowest published airfare at time of booking— or double the difference back!

PLUS—you'll get a $25 voucher to use the first time you book a flight AND 5% cash back on every ticket you buy thereafter through the travel service!

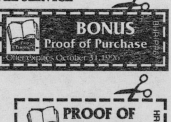

BONUS
Proof of Purchase
Offer expires October 31, 1996

PROOF OF PURCHASE
Offer expires October 31, 1996